Weight Watchers Freestyle

The Only Cookbook You Need In 2018 To Lose Weight Faster and Smarter With Weight Watchers Smart Points Recipes

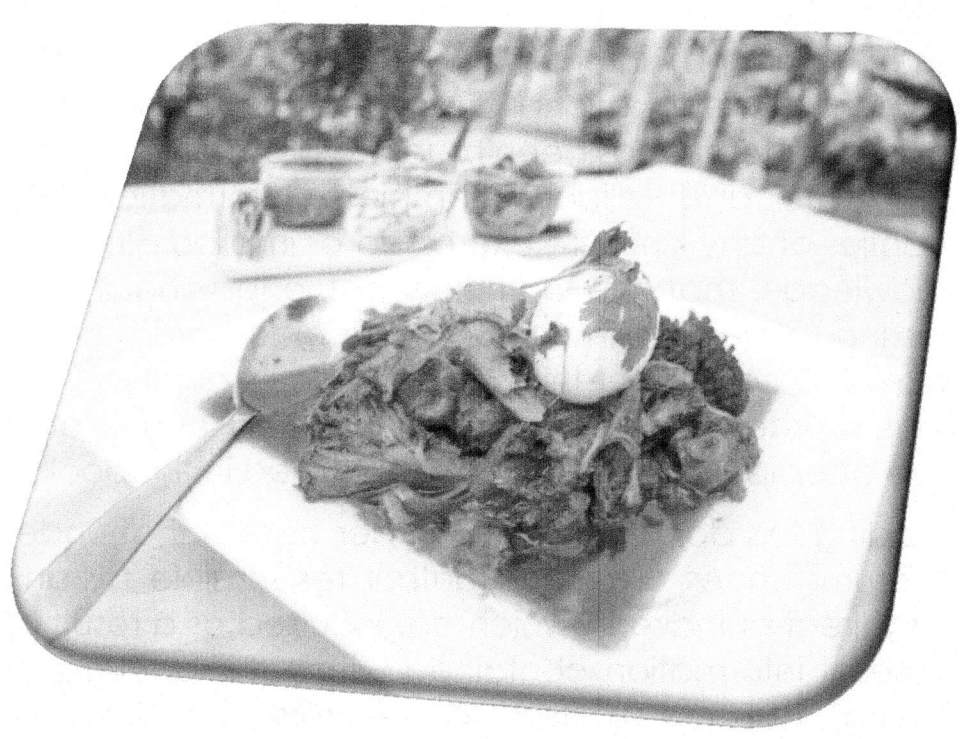

By **Billy Jean**

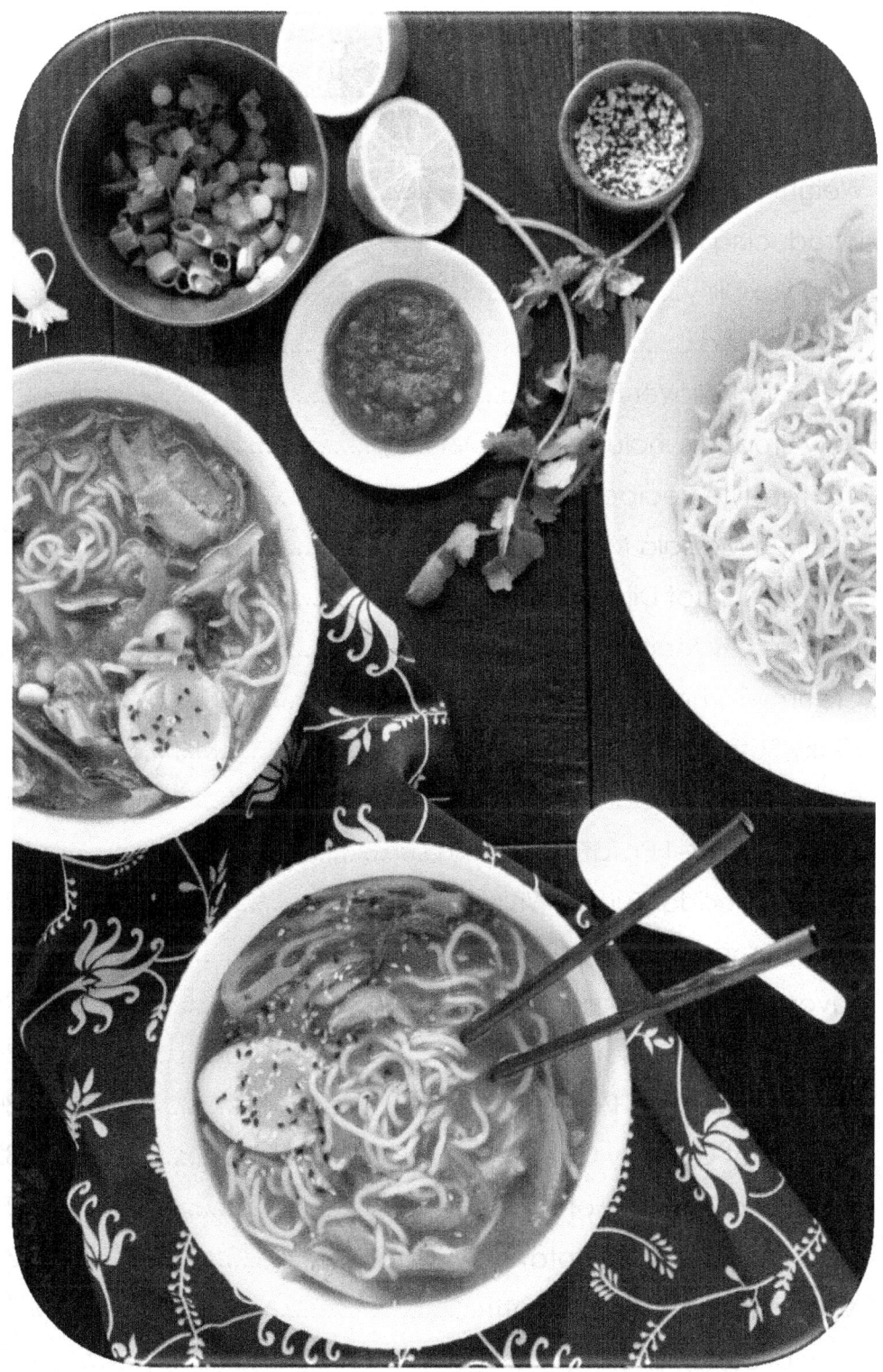

Table of Contents

Introduction

I want to thank you for choosing this book and it may be the best choice you ever made.

Everyone wants to look and feel good, but few are willing to do what it takes to get there. We are all so caught up in our busy lives that we hardly pay any attention to the small habits that make a huge difference. One of the main issues is what we eat and how it affects our bodies.

A large percentage of people around the world are overweight and the struggle to lose weight is real. You have probably heard of tons of different advice on how to lose weight. You might have tried some of those methods as well. But did any of it work for you? The answer to this is probably no. There may be many reasons for this particular failure and it shouldn't leave you frustrated or depressed because you are not the only one facing these problems. Some weight loss methods just take up too much time or effort for you to actually carry them out over a longer period of time. Then there are so many that are just fads and do not really work in reality.

A lot of the quick methods that people try are in fact quite unhealthy for your body and overall health. So we understand why you are stuck in this rut of unsuccessful attempts at losing weight. Here, we will tell you exactly how you can diet and see results. If you keep up with celebrity news or anything related to fitness, you have probably heard of "The Oprah Diet." Well, just like Oprah, we love the Weight Watchers diet too and think it will work for just about anyone who is committed to trying.

The Weight Watchers program is something that has generated a lot of publicity over recent times due to the simple fact that people have seen results and are happy with it. It is not just a diet but a plan through which you make healthy changes in your lifestyle. Ultimately, every small step will help you lose any unwanted weight from your body and gain a much healthier outlook on life.

Weight Watchers will help you make steady progress every day in a way that is not overwhelming or requires you to do things like give up on your favorite food and do strenuous exercise. Instead, it is going to help you steer towards eating healthy food and eat what you like in a more controlled manner so that it doesn't harm your body.

What is Weight Watchers?

If you've ever followed the Weight Watchers plan you'll be all-too-familiar with the Smart Points system, which gives members a daily allowance of points that they can use to construct their meals and snacks. Foods that are higher in sugar and saturated fat are higher in points value, while leaner meats have lower points values and most fruit and veg are zero points (foods that do not cost you any of your points budget).

But now they've introduced Weight Watchers Freestyle (WW Flex as its name in UK) a new program that apparently gives members 'more freedom to enjoy food' by expanding that zero Points food list. And by expand, we mean they've now added foods to it that would have been a higher points value in the old program

Weight Watcher History

Weight Watchers is a great dieting program that is going to help you to lose weight in a safe and effective way. While other diet programs focus on really limiting your calories and telling you what you are allowed to eat and what you should stay away from. While this may work for some people, it can be a big challenge to always be kept away from some of their favorite foods. Plus making food purchases can be difficult on some of the diet plans.

Weight Watchers is going to work a bit differently. It realizes that you have a lot going on in life and you won't be able to sit around and purchase expensive products or go after hard to find ingredients in order to stay healthy. This one is based on the Smart Points that will allow you to eat the foods that work the best for you, but it does reward the healthy foods and discourages the unhealthy foods.

This plan is all about being conscious about your personal eating choices. You will be given a certain amount of points that you are able to use each day, and you get to choose how you use them up. Each of the foods that you choose will have a different point value assigned to it, and you can even make your own recipes and figure out the point values.

This program does allow you to have a bit of cheating throughout the week if you are really craving it or you are not able to resist for a big party. You will find that you can place these into your point's values for the day and still eat them. As long as you are smart about some of the choices that you are making for the rest of the day, these little cheats are not going to ruin the hard work that you put in.

In addition to worrying about the healthy foods that you should consume during the week, there are other parts that come with Weight Watchers. These include going to the meetings and getting more activity into your daily life.

The meetings are a unique part of Weight Watchers that is attributed to some of its success. These meetings are meant to help you be held accountable for the weight that you are supposed to be losing. These usually happen each week and allow you to go in and meet with others in your area who are trying to reach the same goals. You will go in and get weighed, which is a private occurrence, and then you will be able to meet with others to learn new information and get the motivation to help keep you going.

The amount of activity that you do on the Weight Watchers program is going to be important. While this has been changed a bit since the beginning of the program, it is still important to get out there and do a wide variety of activities to ensure that your body is staying healthy and that you are able to lose as much as possible.

The great thing about being on Weight Watchers is that you are able to use it to change your whole lifestyle. This is not some program where you are going to have to work hard at impossible tasks without seeing the great results that you want. Weight Watchers wants you to make a lifestyle change, including eating the right foods, getting activity, and learning the right stuff to keep you on the path you want, in order to really see the results that you want.

Introducing FreeStyle

Based on the successful SmartPoints® system, WW Freestyle offers more than 200 zero Points® foods—including eggs, skinless chicken breast, fish and seafood, corn, beans, peas, and so much more—to multiply your meal and menu possibilities. And it makes life simpler, too: You can forget about weighing, measuring, or tracking those zero Points foods.

Total flexibility

And because we recognize that every day is different—and some days are *really* different (think parties, business travel, holiday open houses....)—we've made your SmartPoints Budget more flexible than ever. Up to 4 unused daily SmartPoints can now roll over into your weekly SmartPoints to give you a bigger "bank" to use whenever and however you like.

How It Works

- For those of you not already familiar with SmartPoints, the SmartPoints system uses the latest nutritional science to make healthy eating as simple as possible. It nudges you toward making healthy choices so eat better and lose weight.

- Every food and drink has a SmartPoints value: a number that is based on calories, protein, sugar and saturated fat. The baseline SmartPoints value is based on the food's calories. Protein lowers the SmartPoints value. Saturated fat and sugar increase the SmartPoints value.

- Every day you get a SmartPoints Budget to spend on any foods you want.

- Your Daily SmartPoints Budget is calculated based on your age, height, weight and gender with a minimum daily value of 23.

- You only need to track the foods that have a SmartPoints value.

- You don't need to weigh, measure or track 0 SmartPoints foods.

- Enjoy a greatly total list of 0 SmartPoints go-to foods at the end of this book.

- Every week you also get a Weekly SmartPoints Budget that you can think of as "overdraft" protection. They are there to use when you go over your Daily SmartPoints budget.

- You can roll over up to four (4) unused Daily SmartPoints into your Weekly SmartPoints. Use them or not as you see fit.

The Daily Rollover Points

With the new Weight Watchers Freestyle plan for 2018, you will be able to roll over up to 4 SmartPoints daily if you do not use them.

I love this idea since it means you could adjust your points to match the natural rhythms and fluctuations of your appetite.

New Products Include Meal Delivery

There's talk of a SmartPoints friendly home meal delivery system similar to those offered by companies like Blue Apron or Hello Fresh, several variations of which are being tested in various regions of the country.

And just at the time this book written, Weight Watchers unveiled its new line of diet wine called Cense, starting with a sauvignon blanc.

Lower in alcohol and calories, the new white wine is "is rich in flavor" but contains only 85 calories per a 5 fluid ounce serving (the equivalent of 3 Weight Watchers SmartPoints), while many other white wines contain about 120 calories (4 SmartPoints) per the same serving size.

Here are some of the latest recipes available so you can try out the Freestyle program

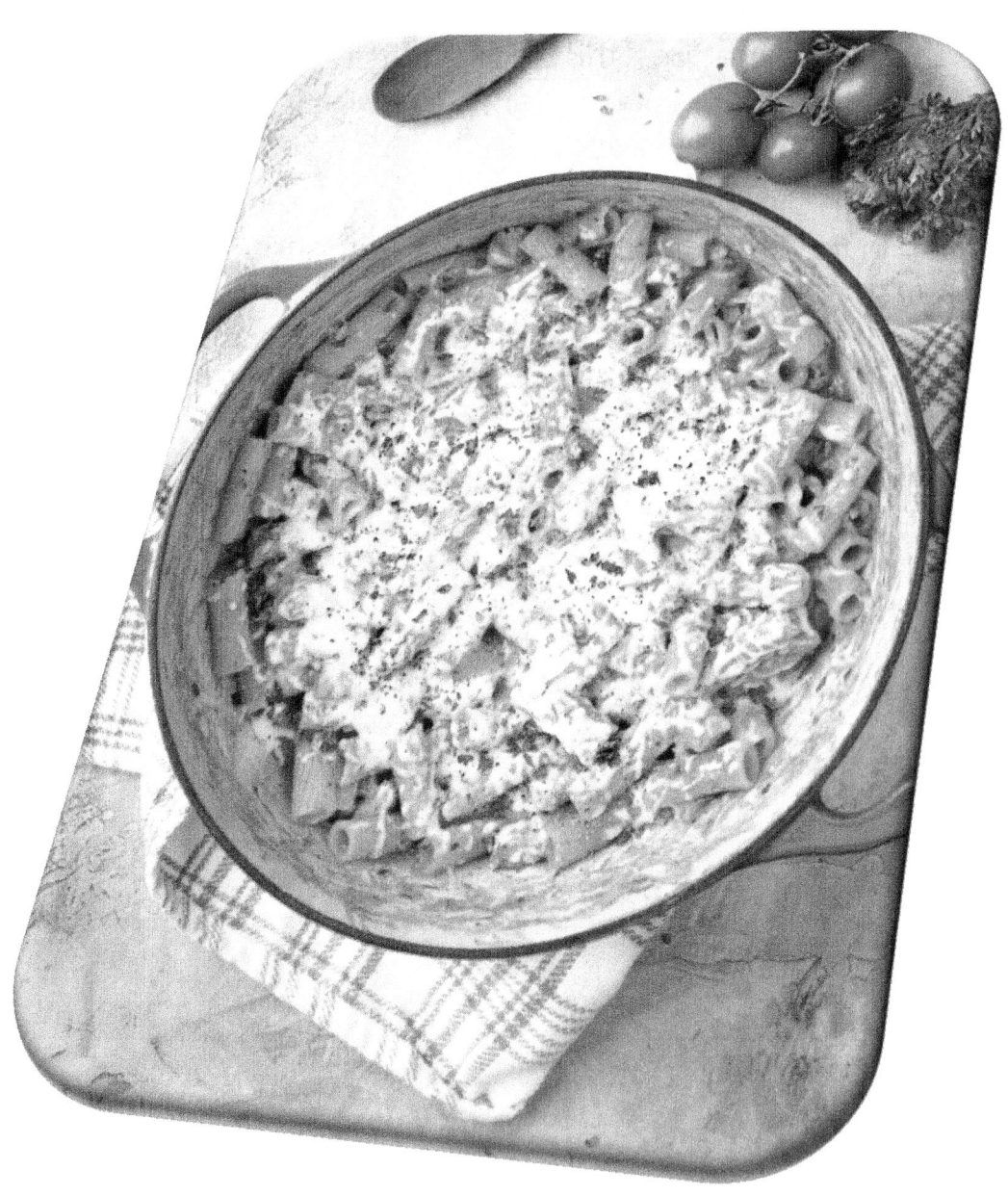

Chicken Marsala MeatBall

5 Free Style Smart Points 248 calories

TOTAL TIME: 30 minutes

INGREDIENTS:

- 8 ounces sliced cremini mushrooms, divided
- 1 pound 93% lean ground chicken
- 1/3 cup whole wheat seasoned or gluten-free bread crumbs
- 1/4 cup grated Pecorino cheese
- 1 large egg, beaten
- 3 garlic cloves, minced
- 2 tablespoons chopped fresh parsley, plus more for garnish
- 1 teaspoon Kosher salt
- Freshly ground black pepper
- 1/2 tablespoon all-purpose flour
- 1/2 tablespoon unsalted butter
- 1/4 cup finely chopped shallots
- 3 ounces sliced shiitake mushrooms
- 1/3 cup Marsala wine
- 3/4 cup reduced sodium chicken broth

DIRECTIONS:

1. Preheat the oven to 400F.
2. Finely chop half of the Cremini mushrooms and transfer to a medium bowl with the ground chicken, breadcrumbs, Pecorino, egg, 1 clove of

the minced garlic, parsley, 1 teaspoon kosher salt and black pepper, to taste.

3. Gently shape into 25 small meatballs, bake 15 to 18 minutes, until golden.

4. In a small bowl whisk the flour with the Marsala wine and broth.

5. Heat a large skillet on medium heat.

6. Add the butter, garlic and shallots and cook until soft and golden, about 2 minutes.

7. Add the mushrooms, season with 1/8 teaspoon salt and a pinch of black pepper, and cook, stirring occasionally, until golden, about 5 minutes.

8. Return the meatballs to the pot, pour the Marsala wine mixture over the meatballs, cover and cook 10 minutes.

9. Garnish with parsley.

NUTRITION INFORMATION

Yield: 5 servings, Serving Size: 5 meatballs with mushrooms

- **Amount Per Serving:**
- **Smart Points: 5, Points +: 6, Calories: 248**
- **Total Fat: 4g, Saturated Fat: 4g**
- **Cholesterol: 121mg, Sodium: 580mg**
- **Carbohydrates: 13g, Fiber: 1.5g, Sugar: 4.5g**
- **Protein: 21g**

Ham & Apricot Dijon Glaze

5 Free Style Smart Points 145 calories

TOTAL TIME: 5 hours

INGREDIENTS:

- 1 (6 to 7 pound) Hickory smoked fully cooked spiral cut ham
- 5 tbsp. apricot preserves
- 2 tablespoons Dijon mustard

DIRECTIONS:

1. Make the glaze: Whisk 4 tablespoons of preserves and mustard together.
2. Place the ham in a 6-quart or larger slow cooker, making sure you can put the lid on. You may have to turn the ham on its side if your ham is too large.
3. Brush the glaze over the ham. Cover and cook on the LOW setting for 4 to 5 hours. Brush the remaining tablespoon of preserves over the ham the 30 minutes.

NUTRITION INFORMATION

Yield: 16, Serving Size: 3 ounces

- **Amount Per Serving:**
- **Smart Points: 5, Points +: 5**
- **Calories: 145, Total Fat: 7g**
- **Saturated Fat: 1.5g, Sodium: 851mg**
- **Carbohydrates: 12g, Fiber: 0g**
- **Sugar: 11g, Protein: 15g**
-

Tasty Turkey Meatball & Veggie

Makes 8 servings.

One serving is 1-1/2 cups soup.

One serving is 5 FreeStyle WW SP.

5 WW FreeStyle SP per serving.

INGREDIENTS

- Cooking spray
- 1 onion, chopped
- 3-4 carrots, sliced or chopped
- 1 cup green beans, cut
- 2 minced garlic cloves
- 1 (24 ounce) package Jennie-O Italian style turkey meatballs
- 2 (14.5 ounce) cans beef or vegetable broth
- 2 (14.5 ounce) diced or Italian stewed tomatoes
- 1-1/2 cups frozen corn
- 1 teaspoon oregano
- 1 teaspoon parsley
- ½ teaspoon basil

INSTRUCTIONS

1. Spray large saucepan or instant pot with cooking spray.
2. Add onions, carrots, green beans and garlic and cook over medium heat 2-3 minutes.
3. Mix in remaining ingredients.

4. If cooking on a stovetop, cover and cook over medium-low heat for 20 minutes, or until meatballs are heated through.

5. -OR-

6. If using an instant pot, press the "soup" button and cook on high pressure for 15 minutes. Vent to release pressure once cooked.

7. -OR-

8. Cook in a slow cooker for 5-6 hours on LOW.

9. Serve warm.

10. Refrigerate or freeze leftovers.

Nutrition Information

- **Serves: 8 servings**
- **Serving size: 1-1/2 cup soup**
- **Calories: 285**
- **Fat: 13 g**
- **Saturated fat: 4 g**
- **Trans fat: 0 g**
- **Carbohydrates: 21 g**
- **Sugar: 9 g**
- **Sodium: 1126 mg**
- **Fiber: 3 g**
- **Protein: 19 g**

Creamy-Tomato-Basil-Soup

Serves: 4

Ingredients

- 1 cup low sodium chicken broth (or vegetable broth if you prefer)
- 1 14 oz. can tomato puree
- 1 cup skim milk
- 4-5 leaves fresh basil
- 3 tsp. olive oil
- 1 stalk celery
- ½ cup onions
- 1 Tbsp. cornstarch
- 1-2 cloves garlic, crushed.
- pepper to taste

Instructions

1. Rough chop onions and celery, transfer them to a food processor or chopper and puree until fine.
2. Heat olive oil in a large pan over medium heat.
3. Add onion and celery mix to pan and sauté until they begin to become translucent.
4. Reduce heat to low and stir in garlic, pepper, chicken stock, and tomato puree, and cornstarch-simmer on low for 5 minutes.
5. Whisk in tomato puree and milk, top with basil leaves, simmer for an additional 10 minutes.
6. Serve topped with a dollop of Greek yogurt or a fresh chopped basil.
7. This makes approximately 4 -1/2 cup servings

Makes 2 large servings

6 PointsPlus per serving

5 SmartPoints per serving on Beyond the Scale, FreeStyle Plan, and Flex Plan

Sticky Buffalo Chicken Tenders

Prep time: 10 mins

Cook time: 15 mins

Total time: 25 mins

Ingredients

- 1 pound boneless skinless chicken breasts, pounded to ½" thickness
- ¼ cup flour
- 3 eggs
- 1 cup Italian Seasoned Panko breadcrumbs
- ½ cup brown sugar
- ⅓ cup Frank's Red Hot Sauce
- ½ teaspoon Garlic Powder
- 3 tablespoons water

Instructions

1. Preheat oven to 425 degrees and spray a baking sheet with non-stick cooking spray or line with silicone baking mats.
2. Cut boneless skinless chicken breasts into strips or chunks (we find chunks hold coating better).
3. Add the chicken into a large Ziploc bag that contains just the flour. Shake to coat.
4. Place Panko breadcrumbs into a shallow bowl. In another shallow bowl, whisk eggs until combined well.
5. Dip flour coated chicken into eggs, then into Panko breadcrumbs to coat.

6. Place coated chicken on the prepared baking sheet. Spray tops with non-stick cooking spray.

7. Bake for 15 minutes for nuggets or 20 minutes for strips or until chicken is browned and cooked through.

8. While chicken is in the oven, you will make your sauce mixture.

9. In a medium saucepan, bring the brown sugar, garlic powder, water and Frank's red hot sauce to a boil. Remove from heat and stir well.

10. When chicken is cooked through, remove from the oven and toss with sauce. This will just coat the chicken.

Makes 6 Servings

7 PointsPlus per Serving

8 SmartPoints per Serving on Beyond the Scale

5 SmartPoints per Serving on FreeStyle or Flex Plan

Garlic Roasted Garbanzo Beans

Prep time: 5 mins
Cook time: 45 mins
Total time: 50 mins
Ingredients

- 1 can garbanzo beans (chickpeas)
- 1 tablespoon olive oil
- 1 teaspoon salt
- 1 teaspoon garlic powder
- ½ teaspoon paprika

Instructions

1. Preheat oven to 375° Fahrenheit.
2. Line a baking sheet with a silicone baking mat or parchment paper.
3. Drain and rinse the garbanzo beans.
4. Pat garbanzo beans dry, pour into a large bowl.
5. Toss with olive oil, salt, garlic powder, and paprika until all are well coated.
6. Spread evenly over baking sheet.
7. Bake at 375° for 20 minutes. Turn chickpeas so they are evenly roasted (use a spatula to flip them or simply stir around but make sure they are in an even layer).
8. Place back in the oven at 375° for additional 25 minutes.
9. Allow the roasted garbanzo beans to cool before storing in an airtight container for snacking.

Makes approximately 3 servings
5 SmartPoints per 1/2 cup on Beyond the Scale, FreeStyle, and Flex Plan

Roasted Sweet Potato Side Dish

Prep time: 5 mins

Cook time: 25 mins

Total time: 30 mins

Ingredients

- 2 Medium Sweet Potatoes
- ½ teaspoon salt
- Non-Stick Cooking Spray

Instructions

1. Preheat oven to 400 degrees.
2. Line baking sheet with silicone baking mat or spray with non-stick spray.
3. Clean sweet potatoes, and peel if desired. We usually leave the skin intact. Remove any blemishes or eyes if needed.
4. Slice sweet potatoes into ¼" thick medallions
5. Place sweet potatoes in a single layer on prepared baking sheet.
6. Sprinkle the tops lightly with salt.
7. Bake at 400 degrees for 15 minutes. Turn sweet potato medallions over and bake additional 10 minutes.

This recipe makes 4 servings.

Each serving is approximately 1/2 sweet potato.

4 PointsPlus per serving

5 SmartPoints per serving on Beyond the Scale

5 SmartPoints per serving on FreeStyle Plan or Flex Plan

Apple Cheddar Turkey Wraps

Yield: 1 WRAP

INGREDIENTS:

- 1 Flatout Light Original Flatbread
- 1-2 leaves green leaf lettuce, torn
- 2 oz. thinly sliced deli turkey
- 1 oz. sliced 50% reduced fat sharp cheddar cheese
- 1 ½ teaspoons apple cider vinegar
- ½ teaspoon canola oil
- ½ teaspoon honey
- A pinch of salt and pepper
- ¼ cup matchstick-sliced apple pieces (slice apple into thin, short sticks)
- 1/3 cup coleslaw mix (just the shredded veggies, undressed)

DIRECTIONS:

1. Lay the Flatout flatbread on a clean, dry surface and lay the torn lettuce down the center of the flatbread going the long way (starting at the rounded end and spreading down the length of the flatbread to the other rounded end). You can leave a bit of space at each end as you'll be folding them over, and you do not need to cover the whole flatbread, just an area down the middle. Top the lettuce with the sliced deli turkey and the cheddar cheese. *Make sure to leave an inch or so of room at each end.*

2. In a small mixing bowl, combine the vinegar, oil, honey, salt and pepper and stir until well

combined. Add the apples and coleslaw and stir to coat. Lay the apple/coleslaw mixture on top of the other ingredients layered on the wrap.

3. Fold in the rounded ends of the flatbread over the filling. Then fold one of the long edges over the filling and continue to roll until the wrap is completely rolled up. Cut in half and serve.

WEIGHT WATCHERS FREESTYLE SMARTPOINTS:
7 per wrap (SP *calculated using the recipe builder on weightwatchers.com*)

WEIGHT WATCHERS POINTS PLUS:
7 per wrap (*P+ calculated using a Weight Watchers brand PointsPlus calculator and the nutrition information below*)

NUTRITION INFORMATION:
277 calories, 26 g carbs, 8 g sugars, 9 g fat, 3 g saturated fat, 28 g protein, 10 g fiber

Pizza Lasagna Roll-Ups

Yield: 8 PIECES
INGREDIENTS:
- 8 uncooked lasagna noodles
- 15 oz. can tomato sauce
- 1 cup pizza sauce
- ½ teaspoon Italian seasoning
- 1 lb. uncooked hot Italian poultry sausage, casings removed if present (I used Wegmans patties, you can use chicken or turkey sausage)
- 2 oz. turkey pepperoni, chopped (reserve 8 slices un-chopped for topping)
- 1 (15 oz.) container fat free Ricotta cheese
- 1 (10 oz.) package frozen chopped spinach, thawed and squeezed until dry

- 1 large egg
- 2 oz. 2% shredded Mozzarella cheese

DIRECTIONS:

1. Pre-heat the oven to 350. Lightly mist a 9×13 baking dish with cooking spray and set aside.
2. Boil and salt a large pot of water and cook lasagna noodles according to package instructions. Drain and rinse with cold water. Lay noodles flat on a clean dry surface and set aside.
3. In a mixing bowl, combine the tomato sauce, pizza sauce and Italian seasoning and stir together. Set aside.
4. Place the sausage in a large skillet over medium heat and cook until browned, breaking the meat up into small pieces as it cooks. When the sausage is cooked through, add the chopped pepperoni and 1/3 cup of the tomato sauce mixture and stir to combine. Remove from heat.
5. In a mixing bowl, combine the ricotta cheese, spinach and egg and stir until well combined. Spoon 1/3 cup of the cheese mixture onto each lasagna noodle and spread across the surface leaving a little room (about ½") at the far end with no toppings. Top the cheese layer on each noodle with the meat mixture from step four, evenly dividing the meat between the noodles. Starting with one end (not the one with space at the end), roll the noodle over the filling until it becomes a complete roll. Repeat with all noodles.
6. Spoon ½ cup of the tomato sauce mixture into the prepared baking dish and spread across the bottom. Place the lasagna rolls seam down in the dish and spoon or pour the remaining sauce over top. Sprinkle the Mozzarella over the top of the rolls

and place a pepperoni on each one. Cover the dish with aluminum foil and bake for 40 minutes.

WEIGHT WATCHERS FREESTYLE SMARTPOINTS:

7 per serving (*SP calculated using the recipe builder on weightwatchers.com*)

WEIGHT WATCHERS POINTS PLUS:

7 per serving (*PP calculated using a PointsPlus calculator and the nutrition information below*)

NUTRITION INFORMATION:

289 calories, 31 g carbs, 9 g sugars, 8 g fat, 2 g saturated fat, 24 g protein, 4 g fiber

Savory Chicken Dump Soup

3 FreeStyle Smart Points per serving (approximately 12 servings / 1 cup each)

Ingredients:

- 1 pound (approx. 3-4) raw skinless boneless chicken thighs
- 1 pkg Trader Joe's frozen Multigrain Blend with Vegetables (if you don't have a TJ's first of all bless your heart.
- Second find another frozen mix with some similar combo to this: cooked grain barley, corn, spelt [wheat], whole rice ermes variety [red], whole rice ribe variety, whole rice-venus variety [black], salt), peas, carrots, water, zucchini, vinegar, extra virgin olive oil, onion, sugar, salt, pepper and totaling no more than 17 SP for the entire bag
- 2 cups (one small package) shredded cabbage
- 1 cup (one small carton fresh or one can) sliced mushrooms any type
- 6 cups water
- 2 tsp dry Italian seasoning

Directions

1. This first part I prep ahead and have on hand in the freezer for easy dumping. If you are anxious to try this right away though there is no need to wait! Just plan a little extra time so your family and friends don't pass out smelling all that yumminess while they stalk you in the kitchen with empty bowls in hand.
2. Add all of the chicken and 1/2 the water to a tall stock pot.
3. Bring everything to a boil for 10 minutes. Reduce to a heavy simmer (not boiling, but bubbling vigorously) and cover loosely with aluminum foil. Let simmer for approximately an hour.
4. Remove one thigh and test with a meat thermometer. If the internal temp is not at least 150 (you want 165 when everything is done!) return and continue simmering for 15 minute intervals until chicken is completely done. If you are making this for prep, remove from heat and allow to cool.
5. Pull chicken apart with two forks to shred or use a hand mixer to "shred" (I haven't used the hand mixer method but I want to try it!).
6. Return to the broth you have just made and then transfer all to a freezer safe container. If you are using immediately return everything to the stock pot and go to the next step.
7. With your stock and shredded chicken in the stock pot, next dump all of the remaining ingredients and stir.
8. Bring back up to a low boil for 10 minutes, then reduce heat and simmer for 30-45 minutes
9.

Zero Points Bean Soup:

0 WW Freestyle Smart Points (12 approximately 1 cup servings)

Ingredients:

- 2 cans white beans (rinsed and drained)
- 2 cans Lima beans (rinsed and drained)
- 2 cans corn kernels drained
- 1 carton low sodium vegetable broth
- 12 slices Canadian Bacon chopped into small pieces
- Season to taste,

Directions:

1. Dump all ingredients into a large crockpot.
2. Stir gently to evenly mix ingredients.
3. Cook on low 6-8 hours. This is zero points…you have enough left for cornbread!

Freestyle Chicken Parmesan

4 Free Style Smart Points 251 calories

TOTAL TIME: 30 minutes

Chicken Parmesan comes out great in the Air Fryer, no need to use so much oil!

INGREDIENTS:

• 2 (about 8 oz. each) chicken breast, fat trimmed, sliced in half to make 4
• 6 tbsp. seasoned breadcrumbs (I used whole wheat, you can use gluten-free)
• 2 tbsp. grated Parmesan cheese
• 1 tbsp. butter, melted (or olive oil)

- 6 tbsp. reduced fat mozzarella cheese
- 1/2 cup marinara
- cooking spray

DIRECTIONS:

1. Preheat the air fryer 360F° for 9 minutes. Spray the basked lightly with spray.

2. Combine breadcrumbs and parmesan cheese in a bowl. Melt the butter in another bowl.

3. Lightly brush the butter onto the chicken, then dip into breadcrumb mixture.

4. When the air fryer is ready, place 2 pieces in the basket and spray the top with oil.

5. Cook 6 minutes, turn and top each with 1 tbsp. sauce and 1 1/2 tbsp. of shredded mozzarella cheese.

6. Cook 3 more minutes or until cheese is melted.

7. Set aside and keep warm, repeat with the remaining 2 pieces.

NUTRITION INFORMATION

Yield: 4 servings, Serving Size: 1 piece

- **Amount Per Serving:**
- **Smart Points: 4, Points +: 6**
- **Calories: 251, Total Fat: 9.5g**
- **Saturated Fat: g, Sodium: mg**
- **Carbohydrates: 14g**
- **Fiber: 1.5g, Sugar: 0g, Protein: 31.5g**
-

Instant Pot Garlicky Cuban Pork

5 Free Style Smart Points 213 calories

TOTAL TIME: 80 minutes plus marinade time

Tender shredded pork, marinated in garlic, cumin, grapefruit and lime and cooked in the pressure cooker is perfect to serve over a bed of rice, cauliflower rice or with tortillas and salsa and avocados for taco night.

INGREDIENTS:

- 3 lb. boneless pork shoulder blade roast, lean, all fat removed
- 6 cloves garlic
- juice of 1 grapefruit (about 2/3 cup)
- juice of 1 lime
- 1/2 tablespoon fresh oregano
- 1/2 tablespoon cumin
- 1 tablespoon kosher salt
- 1 bay leaf
- lime wedges, for serving
- chopped cilantro, for serving
- hot sauce, for serving
- tortillas, optional for serving
- salsa, optional for serving

DIRECTIONS:

1. PRESSURE COOKER: Cut the pork in 4 pieces and place in a bowl.
2. In a small blender or mini food processor, combine garlic, grapefruit juice, lime juice, oregano, cumin and salt and blend until smooth.
3. Pour the marinade over the pork and let it sit room temperature 1 hour or refrigerated as long as overnight.
4. Transfer to the pressure cooker, add the bay leaf, cover and cook high pressure 80 minutes. Let the pressure release naturally.

5. Remove pork and shred using two forks.
6. Remove liquid from pressure cooker, reserving then place the pork back into pressure cooker. Add about 1 cup of the liquid (jus) back, adjust the salt as needed and keep warm until you're ready to eat.

1. SLOW COOKER: Cut the pork in 4 pieces and place in a bowl.
2. In a small blender or mini food processor, combine garlic, grapefruit juice, lime juice, oregano, cumin and salt and blend until smooth.
3. Pour the marinade over the pork and let it sit room temperature 1 hour or refrigerated as long as overnight.
4. Transfer to the slow cooker, add the bay leaf, cover and cook low 8 hours.
5. Remove pork and shred using two forks.
6. Remove liquid from slow cooker, reserving then place the pork back into slow cooker. Add about 1 cup of the liquid (jus) back, adjust the salt as needed and keep warm until you're ready to eat.

NUTRITION INFORMATION
Yield: 10 servings, Serving Size: a little over 3 oz.
- **Amount Per Serving:**
- **Smart Points: 5, Points +: 5**
- **Calories: 213, Total Fat: 9.5g**
- **Saturated Fat: 0g, Sodium: 440.5mg**
- **Carbohydrates: 2.5g, Fiber: 0.5g**
- **Sugar: 1.5g, Protein: 26.5g**

Scalloped, Ham & Potatoes

Prep Time: 45 m, **Cook Time:** 7 h, **Total Time:** 7 hrs. 45 m

Slow cooker scalloped potatoes and ham, a comforting classic dish made lighter your whole family will love.

Delicious Scalloped Potatoes & Ham

Ingredients

- 8 cups peeled and thinly sliced potatoes (8 to 10 medium)
- Salt and pepper to taste
- 1 medium onion, sliced thin (about 1 cup)
- 1-1/2 cups cubed cooked ham
- 1 cup grated low-fat cheddar cheese
- 1 can (10-1/2 ounces) low-fat cream of mushroom soup (I used Campbell's Healthy Request)
- Paprika

Instructions

1. Ideal slow cooker size: 4- to 5-Quart.
2. Grease your slow cooker with nonstick cooking spray.
3. Put half the sliced potatoes in the bottom of your slow cooker, spreading them out evenly. Sprinkle with salt and pepper to taste.
4. Sprinkle evenly with half the onion, ham and cheese.
5. Repeat the layers one more time (potatoes, salt and pepper, onion, ham, cheese).

6. Pour the soup into a small bowl and stir it until it gets nice and creamy. Spread it over the top of the ingredients in the slow cooker.

7. Cover and cook on LOW for 6 to 8 hours, or until the potatoes and onions are tender when pierced with a fork.

8. Just before serving, sprinkle with a little paprika.

Nutrition Facts

Weight Watchers PointsPlus: *6

Weight Watchers SmartPoints: *7

Amount per Serving (1 cup)

Calories 249Calories from Fat 30

% Daily Value*

Total Fat 3.3g**5%**

Total Carbohydrates 40.4g**13%**

Dietary Fiber 5.7g**23%**

Protein 14.3g**29%**

* Percent Daily Values are based on a 2000 calorie diet.

Marinara Spinach manicotti

7 Free Style Smart Points 277 calories

COOK TIME: 25 minutes

INGREDIENTS:

- 16 homemade crespelles
- 15 oz. part skim ricotta cheese (I use Polly-O)
- 2 cups shredded part-skim mozzarella cheese (reserve 1/2 cup) Polly-O
- 1 large egg
- 10 oz. package frozen spinach, thawed and squeezed really well

- 1/4 cup grated Parmesan Regianno
- 1/2 teaspoon kosher salt
- black pepper, to taste
- 2 1/2 cups jarred marinara

DIRECTIONS:

1. Start by making the crespelles.
2. Preheat oven to 375°F.
3. In a large bowl, combine ricotta, 1-1/2 cups of the mozzarella, egg, spinach, parmesan cheese, 1/2 teaspoon salt and pepper.
4. Fill each crespelle with 1/4 cup spinach filling and roll.
5. In a large baking dish, (or two smaller dishes) pour 1 cup of sauce on the bottom of the dish.
6. Place rolled manicotti seem side down onto baking dish. Top with 1 1/2 cups more sauce and remaining mozzarella cheese.
7. Cover with foil and bake about about 25 minutes, until hot and bubbling, and the cheese is melted.

NUTRITION INFORMATION

Yield: 8 servings, Serving Size: 2 manicotti

- **Amount Per Serving:**
- **Smart Points: 7,**
- **Points +: 7,**
- **Calories: 277**
- **Total Fat: 12.5g**
- **Saturated Fat: 6g**
- **Sodium: 698mg**
- **Carbohydrates: 20g**
- **Fiber: 3g**
- **Sugar: 5g**
- **Protein: 22.5g**

Peanut Butter Overnight Oats

Prep time: 5 mins

Total time: 5 mins

Makes 1 Serving 6 PointsPlus per serving

7 SmartPoints per Serving on Beyond the Scale

7 SmartPoints per Serving on FreeStyle Plan or Flex Plan

Ingredients

- ½ cup old-fashioned oats
- ¾ cup milk or almond milk
- 1 tablespoon peanut butter
- 1 tablespoon sugar-free jam

Instructions

1. Combine the oats, almond milk, and PB2 powder in a bowl and mix well.
2. Place bowl in the refrigerator for 1 hour and allow to set.
3. In an 8 oz. mason jar alternate a heaping spoon of oatmeal and a small spoon of sugar-free jam to the top.
4. Replace lid/ring on jar and place in refrigerator overnight.
5. In the morning stir gently before serving.

Makes 1 Serving

6 PointsPlus per serving

7 SmartPoints per Serving on Beyond the Scale

7 SmartPoints per Serving on FreeStyle Plan or Flex Plan

Fat Free Pimento Chile Chicken

Ingredients:

- 2 ½ c. cooked, chopped chicken breast (chopped into about 1/2" cubes
- ½ c. fat free chicken broth
- 1 ½ c. 98% fat free cream of mushroom soup (I use Campbell's)
- 1 ½ c. Healthy Request Condensed cream of chicken soup
- 1 4-oz. jar pimentos, drained (1/2 c.)
- 2 4-oz. cans Hatch green chiles, chopped and drained (You can add a 3rd can if you're just crazy about chiles like I am.)
- 10 oz. 50% reduced fat sharp cheddar cheese
- 6 oz. of Doritos (by weight) toasted corn tortilla chips, slightly crushed
- Pickled jalapeños, green onions, and/or cherry tomatoes for serving (optional)

Instructions:

1. Mix all ingredients except Doritos and cheese. In a large casserole dish (I use 9" x 13"), layer ½ of chicken mixture, then ½ of cheese, then ½ of the Doritos.
2. Repeat the same layers once more, ending with Doritos on top. Bake at 350° for about 40-45 minutes.
3. Cover top with foil if Doritos begin to brown too much.
4. Serve with pickled jalapeños and/or your favorite salsa.

Weight Watchers Info.

6 points per serving in the new Freestyle plan;
Makes 8 servings.

Delicious Buffalo Chicken Pasta

Prep time: 5 m, Cook time: 35 m, Total time: 40 mins

Ingredients

- 2 cups shredded or cubed chicken
- 1 box penne pasta (12 oz.)
- 8 ounces fat-free cream cheese
- ⅓-1/2 cup Frank's Hot Sauce (this is to taste if you prefer hotter or not)
- 1 package Ranch Seasoning Mix
- ½ cup fat-free sour cream
- 1 cup fat-free cheddar cheese, divided

Instructions

1. Preheat oven to 375 degrees.
2. Cook pasta according to package, drain and set aside
3. Spray a large casserole dish (9x13) with nonstick spray
4. Mix drained pasta with chicken, cream cheese, Frank's sauce, ranch mix, sour cream, and ½ cup cheese until well blended.
5. Pour into casserole dish and spread evenly.
6. Top with remaining cheese
7. Bake for 18-20 minutes or until heated through and cheese has melted.

Makes 8 Servings
Each serving is 1 1/2 cups
7 SmartPoints per serving
6 SmartPoints on FreeStyle Plan or Flex Plan

Italian Creamy Chicken Pasta Recipe

Prep time: 10 m, Cook time: 15 m, Total time: 25 mins

Ingredients

- 1 pound boneless skinless chicken breast, cubed
- 16oz box penne pasta
- 2 cups chicken stock (or water)
- 2 Roma tomatoes, diced
- ½ red onion, diced
- 1 cup mushrooms, diced
- 2 cloves garlic, minced (can use equivalent garlic powder if you prefer)
- 2 teaspoons Italian seasonings
- 1 cup low-fat part-skim mozzarella cheese, shredded
- ½ cup fat-free cream cheese

Instructions

1. Add all ingredients to Instant Pot liner, except for cheeses.
2. Mix well so that pasta is covered in liquid and everything is well combined.
3. Place lid and set to seal.
4. Set to high pressure (manual) for 9 minutes. Once done, allow to NPR (natural pressure release) for 5 minutes.
5. Once pressure has released, remove the lid and stir in cheeses until well combined and melted.
6. Serve with additional Parmesan or parsley as desired.

Makes 8 servings (1 1/2 cup per serving)

10 PointsPlus

6 SmartPoints on FreeStyle or Flex Plans

8 SmartPoints per Serving on Beyond the Scale

One Pot Slow & Pressure Cook recipes:

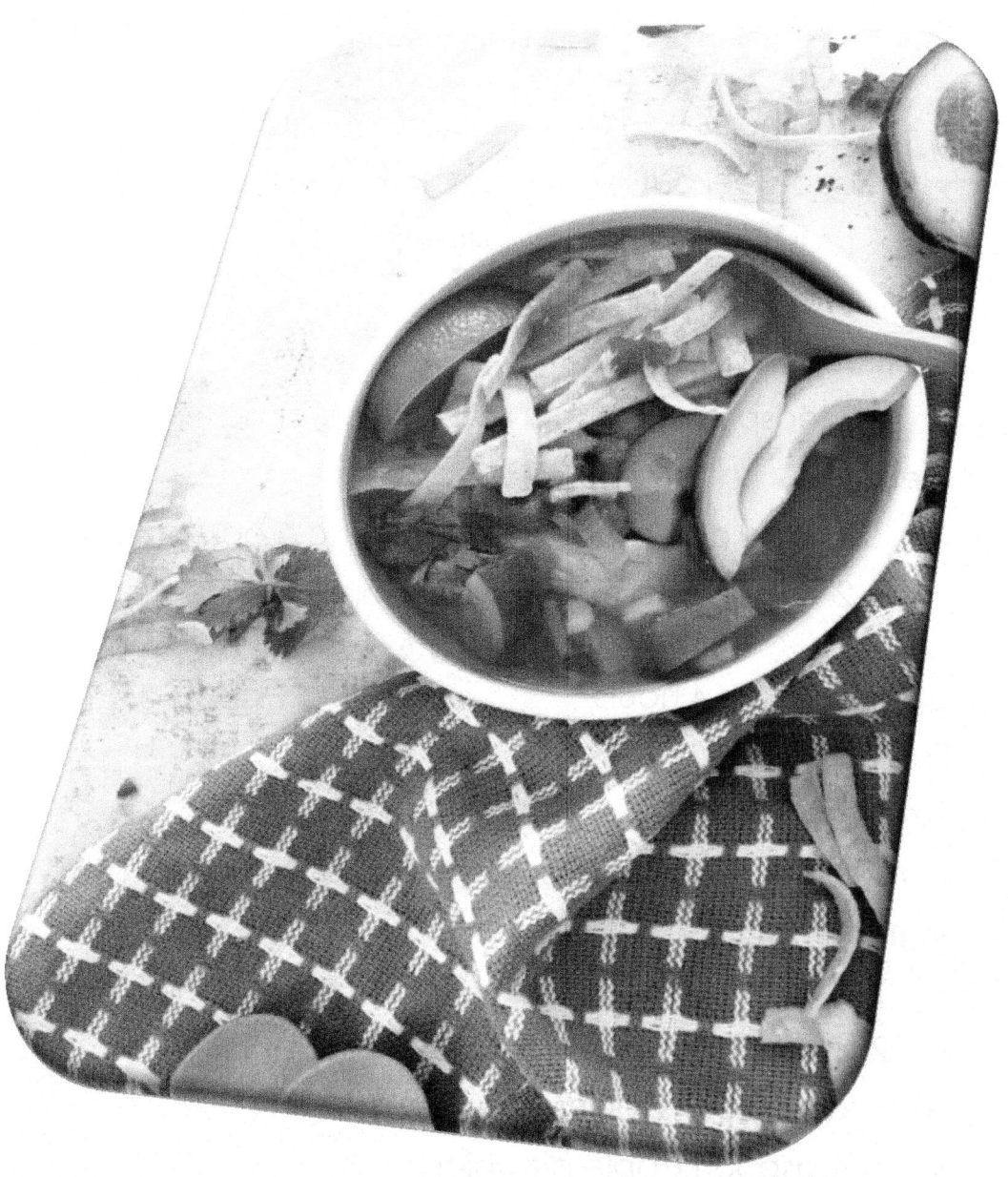

Tasty Pumpkin Oatmeal

Cooking time: 8 hours

Serves: 4

Smart points: 7

Ingredients:

- 1 ½ cups pie pumpkin or sugar pumpkin, peeled, deseeded, cubed
- ¼ cup honey
- ¾ cup steel cut oats, uncooked
- ½ teaspoon ground cinnamon
- ¼ teaspoon salt or to taste
- 3 cups water
- 1/8 teaspoon nutmeg, grated or ground

Method:

1. Add all the ingredients into the crock-pot and stir.
2. Cover and cook on Low for 7-8 hours.

Baked Sliced Apples

Cooking time: 4 hours

Serves: 3

Smart points: 4

Calories: 69, Carb 16 g, Sugar 12 g, Fat 1g, Protein 0 g

Ingredients:

- 1 ¾ cups cooking apple, peeled, cored, thickly slice
- 2 tablespoons granular splenda
- 2 tablespoons raisins, seedless
- ¾ teaspoon apple pie spice

- ½ tablespoon reduced calorie margarine
- Butter flavored cooking spray

Method:

1. Spray the inside of the slow cooker with cooking spray
2. Add all the ingredients except margarine and stir. Place margarine on top.
3. Cover and cook on 'Low' for 4 hours.

Delicious Crust-less Apple Pie

Cooking time: 4-5 hours

Serves: 4

Smart points: 9

Calories: 174, Carbohydrate – 47g, Fiber – 8 g, Sugar – 35 g, Fat – 1 g, Protein – 1 g

Ingredients:

- ½ cup splenda
- 1 tablespoon ground cinnamon or to taste
- 5 large Granny Smith apples, peeled, cored, chopped into chunks
- ½ cup water

Method:

1. Place apples in the crock-pot. Mix together rest of the ingredients and pour over the apples.
2. Cover and cook on 'Low' for 4-5 hours. Stir occasionally.
3. Serve warm with ice cream or whipped cream if desired.

Slow Cook Lasagna

Cooking time: 4-6 hours

Serves: 3

Smart points: 11

Calories: 360, Carbohydrate –31 g, Fiber – 4 g, Sugar – 8 g, Fat – 14 g, Saturated fat – 7 g, Protein – 28 g,

Ingredients:

- ½ pound lean ground beef
- 7.5 ounces tomato sauce
- 1 clove garlic, minced
- 14 ounces canned crushed tomatoes
- 1 medium onion, chopped
- ¼ teaspoon red pepper flakes
- Salt to taste
- ¼ teaspoon dried basil
- ½ teaspoon dried oregano
- ¾ cup low fat mozzarella cheese, cubed
- ½ cup part skim ricotta cheese
- ¼ cup parmesan cheese, shredded
- 3 lasagna noodles, broken in half

Method:

1. Place a skillet over medium high heat. Add beef, onion and garlic and sauté until brown. Break it simultaneously as it cooks.

2. Add tomatoes, tomato sauce, salt, oregano, basil and red pepper flakes and stir. Simmer for 3-4 minutes. Remove from heat.

3. Mix together in a bowl ricotta and ½ cup mozzarella cheese.

4. Pour 1/3 of the cooked sauce into the slow cooker. Place 3 halves of the lasagna noodles over it. Sprinkle half the cheese mixture.

5. Repeat the above layer once. Finally pour the remaining 1/3 of the cooked sauce over it.

6. Cover and cook on 'Low' for 4-6 hours.

7. Mix together in a bowl ¼ cup mozzarella and Parmesan.

8. When the cook time is over, sprinkle the cheese mixture over it. Cover and let it sit for 10 minutes before serving.

Chicken Stroganoff

Cooking time: 6 - 7 hours

Serves: 3

Smart points: 7

Calories: 216, Carbohydrate – 15 g, Fiber – 0 g, Sugar – 6 g, Fat – 8 g,

Saturated fat – 3 g, Protein – 20 g,

Ingredients:

- 5.5 ounces 98% fat free cream of chicken soup or cream of mushroom soup

- 2/3 ounce onion soup mix

- ½ pound frozen chicken breast, skinless

- 8 ounces fat free sour cream

Method:

1. Place the chicken at the bottom of the slow cooker. Mix together rest of the ingredients in a bowl and pour over and around the chicken.

2. Cover and cook on 'Low' for 6-7 hours.

Delicious Beef Stroganoff

Yields: 4

Cooking time: 25 minutes

Preparation time: 10 minutes

Nutritional Information per Serving:

Calories: 279, SmartPoints: 8

Ingredients

- 6-ounces sirloin steak, fat-trimmed and cut into strips
- 1 ½ cup mushrooms, sliced
- ½ cup onion, chopped
- 3 cloves of garlic, chopped
- 1 cup beef broth
- ¼ cup tomato sauce
- 3 tablespoon sherry wine
- ¾ tablespoon Worcestershire sauce
- ¼ teaspoon salt
- ¼ teaspoon pepper
- 1/3 cup sour cream
- 1 cup dry medium egg noodles
- 2 teaspoon fresh parsley, chopped

Instructions

1.   Press the Sauté button and cook the steak for 3 minutes. Add the mushroom, onion, and garlic and cook for another two minutes.

2.   Pour in the broth, tomato sauce, sherry wine, and Worcestershire sauce. Season with salt and pepper to taste.

3.   Close the lid and press the manual button. Cook on high for 25 minutes.

4.   Do quick pressure release.

5.   Once the lid is open, press the sauté button and add the sour cream and noodles.

6.   Cook for 7 to 10 more minutes until the noodles are done.

7.   Garnish with parsley.

Chipotles Barbecue Beef

Yields: 9

Cooking time: 40 minutes

Preparation time:

Nutritional Information per Serving:

Calories: 153, SmartPoints: 3

Ingredients

- ½ medium onion, chopped
- 5 cloves of garlic, minced
- 1 tablespoon ground cumin
- 1 lime, juiced
- 4 tablespoon chipotles in adobo sauce
- 1 tablespoon ground oregano

- ½ teaspoon ground cloves
- 1 cup water
- 3-pounds beef eye or round roast with fat trimmed
- 2 ½ teaspoon salt
- Black pepper to taste
- 1 teaspoon oil
- 3 bay leaves

Instructions

1.   Place onion, garlic, cumin, lime juice, chipotles, oregano, and cloves in a blender. Add water and blend until smooth.

2.   Season the beef with salt and pepper.

3.   Press the Sauté button on the Instant Pot and heat the oil.

4.   Add the beef and cook for 5 minutes until it turns brown on all sides.

5.   Add the puree and bay leaves.

6.   Close the lid and cook for 35 minutes.

7.   Do quick pressure release.

8.   Remove the beef and shred using a fork. Discard the bay leaves.

9.   Return the shredded meat into the pot and adjust the seasoning.

Sweet and Sour Chicken

Yields: 4

Cooking time: 10 minutes

Preparation time: 5 minutes

Nutritional Information per Serving:

Calories: 206, SmartPoints: 7

Ingredients

- Cooking spray to coat the inner pot
- 1 pound boneless chicken breast
- ¼ teaspoon onion powder
- ¼ teaspoon garlic powder
- 5 ounce sweet and sour sauce
- 1 tablespoon brown sugar
- 8-ounces pineapple chunks
- 16 ounces of mixed frozen vegetables

Instructions

1. Coat the inner pot of your Instant Pot with cooking spray.
2. Press the Sauté button and add the chicken, onion powder, and garlic powder.
3. Add in the sweet and sour sauce, brown sugar, and pineapple chunks with juice.
4. Stir in the frozen vegetables.
5. Close the lid and press the manual button. Cook on high pressure for 7 minutes.
6. Do quick release to open the lid.

Tomato Spinach Soup

Cooking time: 4 hours

Serves: 4

Smart points: 2

Calories: 43, Carbohydrate – 9 g, Fiber – 3 g, Sugar – 5 g, Fat –0 g, Protein – 2 g

Ingredients:

- 1 medium carrot, chopped
- 5 ounces baby spinach
- 1 medium stalk celery, chopped
- 1 clove garlic, minced
- 1 medium onion, chopped
- 2 cups vegetable broth
- Salt to taste
- Pepper to taste
- ½ teaspoon dried oregano
- ½ tablespoon dried basil
- ¼ teaspoon crushed red pepper flakes
- 14 ounces canned diced tomatoes
- 1 bay leaf

Method:

1. Add all the ingredients into the slow cooker.
2. Clover and set on High for 5 hours.
3. Discard bay leaf and stir.
4. Ladle into soup bowls and serve.

Provencal Beef Stew

Cooking time: 5-6 hours

Serves: 3

Smart points: 3

Ingredients:

- 1 small onion, chopped
- 7.5 ounces canned pinto beans, drained, rinsed, divided
- 1 cup fresh mushrooms, sliced
- 1 large carrot, sliced
- 1 cup beef broth, divided
- 1 clove garlic, minced
- 8 ounces beef stew meat, chopped into 1 inch pieces
- ¼ teaspoon dried thyme
- ¼ teaspoon dried oregano
- Salt to taste
- Pepper to taste
- Cooking spray

Method:

1. Place a skillet over medium high heat. Spray with cooking spray. Add onion, garlic and mushrooms and sauté for 4-5 minutes. Transfer into the slow cooker.

2. Blend half the pinto beans in a blender adding half the broth. Pour into the slow cooker.

3. Add the remaining beans, carrots, tomatoes, remaining broth, herbs, salt and pepper and stir.

4. Cover and set on 'High' for 5-6 hours.

Tasty Italian Meatloaf

Yields: 4
Cooking time: 25 minutes
Preparation time: 15 minutes

Nutritional Information per Serving:
Calories: 240, SmartPoints: 7

Ingredients
- ¼ cup onion, chopped
- 1 pound lean ground beef
- 2 large egg whites
- ¼ cup seasoned Italian bread crumbs
- ½ cup barbecue sauce, divided

Instructions
1. In a mixing bowl, combine onion, meat, egg whites, and bread crumbs. Season with ¼ of the barbecue sauce.
2. Shape the mixture into a log and place them on parchment paper. Make sure that it will fit inside the Instant Pot.
3. Place a trivet or steam rack in the instant pot and add 1 ½ cups of water.
4. Set the meatloaf on top of the steam rack.
5. Close the lid and press the manual button. Cook on high for 25 minutes.
6. Do quick pressure release to remove the meatloaf.
7. Let it cool for one hour before pouring the remaining sauce on top.
8. You also have an option to broil it in the oven for 15 minutes to achieve browning.

Easy Instant Lasagna

Yields: 6
Cooking time: 20 minutes
Preparation time: 10 minutes

Nutritional Information per Serving:
Calories: 360, SmartPoints: 11

Ingredients

- 1 pound lean ground beef
- 1 clove of garlic, minced
- 1 onion, chopped
- 1 can tomato sauce
- 1 can tomato, crushed
- 1 teaspoon salt
- ½ teaspoon dried basil
- 1 teaspoon dried oregano
- ¼ teaspoon red pepper flakes
- 1 ½ cup low-fat mozzarella cheese, grated
- 1 cup part-skim ricotta cheese
- 6 lasagna noodle
- ½ cup water
- ½ cup parmesan cheese, grated

Instructions

1. Press the Sauté button on the Instant Pot and add the ground beef, garlic and onions. Stir constantly to avoid browning at the bottom and also to break up large pieces of the beef.
2. Add in the tomato sauce and crushed tomatoes. Season with salt, dried basil, oregano, and red pepper flakes. Set aside to assemble the lasagna.
3. Prepare the cheese sauce by mixing the 1 cup of mozzarella with ricotta.
4. Break the lasagna noodles and stir in the pot.
5. Place ¾ cup of the meat mixture at the bottom of the pot then drizzle with the cheese sauce. Add a layer of lasagna noodles. Do this alternately until all ingredients are placed inside the pot. Pour over water.
6. Close the lid and press the manual button. Cook on high for 15 minutes.
7. Do natural release to open the lid.
8. Sprinkle with parmesan cheese for garnish.

Steamed Jalapeno Chicken

Yields: 4

Cooking time: 10 minutes

Preparation time: 8 hours

Nutritional Information per Serving:

Calories: 202, SmartPoints: 5

Ingredients

- ½ cup jalapeno jelly, melted
- ½ cup steak sauce
- 1 teaspoon garlic powder
- 2 tablespoon low-sodium Worcestershire sauce
- 4-ounces boneless chicken breasts, skin removed

Instructions

1. In a bowl, mix together the jalapeno jelly, steak sauce, garlic powder and Worcestershire sauce.
2. Marinate the chicken for at least 8 hours.
3. Remove the chicken from the bag and remove the marinade.
4. Place a steamer inside the Instant Pot and add the chicken pieces. Add 1 cup of water.
5. Close the lid and press the manual button. Cook on high for 10 minutes.
6. Do quick pressure release

Instant Beef Picadillo

Cooking time: 20 minutes

Serves: 3

Smart points: 3

Calories: 207, Carbohydrate – 5 g, Fiber –1 g, Sugar – 3 g, Fat – 8.5 g, Protein – 25 g

Ingredients:

- ¾ pound 93% lean ground beef
- 1 clove garlic, minced
- 1 medium onion, chopped
- ¼ red bell pepper, finely chopped
- 1 small tomato, chopped
- 2 ounces canned tomato sauce
- 1 bay leaf
- Fresh cilantro, chopped to garnish
- 1 tablespoons capers or green olives

Method:

1. Select 'Sauté' option. Add meat. Press 'Adjust' button once. Sauté until meat is brown. Add salt and pepper. Break it simultaneously as it cooks.

2. Add rest of the ingredients and stir.

3. Close the lid. Select 'Manual' option in instant pot or 'High pressure' option in pressure cooker and set the timer for 15 minutes. Let the pressure release naturally.

Instant Italian Pulled Pork

Cooking time: 55 minutes

Serves: 5

Smart points: 1

Calories: 93, Carbohydrate – 6.5 g, Fiber – 0 g, Sugar – 3 g, Fat – 1.5 g, Protein – 11 g

Ingredients:

- 9 ounces pork tenderloin
- 3 cloves garlic, smashed
- 1 teaspoon olive oil
- 14 ounces canned crushed tomatoes
- 1 bay leaf
- 3.5 ounces roasted red peppers from a jar, drained
- Kosher salt to taste
- Pepper to taste
- A handful fresh parsley, chopped
- 1 sprig fresh thyme

Method:

1. Select 'Sauté' option. Add oil. When the oil is heated, add garlic and stir until it turns golden brown. Remove the garlic with a slotted spoon and set aside.

2. Add pork. Sprinkle salt and pepper. Cook until brown on both sides (about 2 minutes per side).

3. Add garlic and rest of the ingredients and stir.

4. Close the lid. Select 'Meat' option for instant pot or 'High pressure' option in pressure cooker with timer set for 45 minutes.

5. Let the pressure release naturally. Discard the bay leaf. Remove the meat with a slotted spoon. When cool enough to handle, shred the pork with a pair of forks.

6. Garnish with parsley and serve over pasta.

Tasty Teriyaki Chicken

Cooking time: 4 hours

Serves: 3

Smart points: 9

Calories: 318, Carbohydrate – 25 g, Fiber – 0 g, Sugar – 24 g, Fat – 5 g, Saturated fat – 1 g, Protein – 43 g,

Ingredients:

• 1 ¼ pounds chicken breast, skinless, boneless, chopped into 2 inch pieces

• ¼ cup honey

• ¼ cup soy sauce

• 2 whole cloves garlic

• 1 teaspoon hot chili sauce

Method:

1. Place the chicken at the bottom of the slow cooker. Mix together rest of the ingredients in a bowl and pour over and around the chicken.

2. Cover and cook on 'Low' for 4 hours. Stir once half way through cooking.

Tasty Beef Burgundy

Cooking time: 5 ½ hours

Serves: 3

Smart points: 13

Calories: 488.8, Carbohydrate – 38.1 g, Fiber – 3.5 g, Sugar – 5.7 g, Fat – 17 g, Saturated fat – 6.2 g, Protein – 41.3 g

Ingredients:

- 1 pound round steak, trimmed of fat, chopped into bite size pieces
- 1 clove garlic, minced
- 1 tablespoon tomato paste
- 1 medium onion, sliced
- 8 ounces frozen small whole onions, thawed, drained
- 5 ounces condensed beef broth, undiluted
- 3 tablespoons all-purpose flour
- ¼ cup red wine
- 4 ounces fresh mushrooms sliced
- ¼ teaspoon dried thyme
- ½ teaspoon salt or to taste
- 1 bay leaf
- Pepper to taste
- 1 ½ cups medium egg noodles, cook according to the instructions on the package
- Cooking spray

Method:

1. Place a skillet over medium heat. Spray with cooking spray. Add beef and sauté until brown. Transfer into the slow cooker.
2. Spray again with cooking spray. Add sliced onions and garlic and sauté until translucent. Add flour and sauté for about a minute.
3. Add broth, wine and tomato paste. Stir constantly until thick. Add whole onions, mushrooms, bay leaf, thyme, pepper and salt and stir. Transfer into the instant pot.
4. Cover and cook on 'High' for an hour. Then switch to 'Low' and cook for 4 ½ hours.
5. When done, discard the bay leaf.
6. Divide the egg noodles in 3 bowls. Ladle beef over it and serve.

Balsamic Pork Roast

Cooking time: 4 hours

Serves: 4

Smart points: 5

Calories: 214, Carbohydrate – 4 g, Fiber – 0 g, Sugar – 3 g, Fat – 12 g, Protein – 21 g

Ingredients:

- 1 pound boneless pork shoulder roast
- ¼ teaspoon red pepper flakes
- ¼ teaspoon garlic powder
- Kosher salt to taste
- 3 tablespoon chicken or vegetable broth
- 2 teaspoons Worcestershire sauce
- 3 tablespoons balsamic vinegar
- ½ tablespoon honey

Method:

1. Sprinkle salt, pepper, red pepper flakes and garlic powder all over the pork and place it in the crock-pot.

2. Mix together rest of the ingredients and pour over the pork.

3. Cover and cook on 'High' for 4 hours or on 'Low' for 8 hours.

4. When done, remove the pork with a slotted spoon. When cool enough to handle, shred with a pair of forks and add it back to the crock-pot.

5. Heat thoroughly and serve.

Tasty Jerk Turkey Soup

Cooking time: 6-7 hours

Serves: 3

Smart points: 4

Calories: 196, Carbohydrate – 18 g, Fiber – 5 g, Sugar – 1 g, Fat – 2 g, Saturated fat – 1 g Protein – 27 g

Ingredients:

- 7.5 ounces canned black beans, drained, rinsed
- 7.5 ounces fire roasted diced tomatoes with green chili pepper with its liquid
- ½ pound turkey breast, chopped into 1 inch pieces
- 1 small onion, chopped
- 1 clove garlic, minced
- ¼ teaspoon ground ginger
- ¼ teaspoon ground allspice
- ¼ teaspoon garlic salt
- Salt to taste
- ¼ teaspoon cayenne pepper
- 2 cups chicken broth
- 1 tablespoon fresh cilantro, chopped
- 2 teaspoons fresh lemon juice

Method:

1. Mix together in a bowl, allspice, cayenne pepper, garlic salt, ginger and a little pepper. Add turkey and toss well. Set aside for a while.
2. Transfer the turkey into a slow cooker. Add remaining ingredients except lemon juice and cilantro and stir.
3. Cover and cook on 'Low' for 6-7 hours or on 'High' for 2 ½ - 3 hours.

Sweet & Sour Chicken

Cooking time: 6-7 hours

Serves: 2

Smart points: 7

Calories: 206, Carbohydrate – 19 g, Fiber – 1 g, Sugar – 5 g, Fat – 3 g,

Saturated fat – 1 g, Protein – 25 g,

Ingredients:

- ½ pound chicken breast, skinless, boneless
- ¼ teaspoon onion powder
- ¼ teaspoon garlic powder
- 2.5 ounces sweet and sour sauce
- 4 ounces canned pineapple chunks with 2-3 tablespoons of its juice
- 8 ounces stir fry vegetables
- ½ tablespoon brown sugar
- Cooking spray

Method:

1. Spray the inside of the crock-pot with cooking spray.
2. Place the chicken in the crock-pot. Season the chicken with garlic powder and onion powder,
3. Mix together rest of the ingredients except vegetables and pour over the chicken.
4. Cover and cook on 'Low' for 6-7 hours.

Cheeseburger Soup

Cooking time: 2 hours

Serves: 4

Smart points: 7

Calories: 208, Carb 7 g, Sugar 3 g, Fat 10 g, Protein –22 g

Ingredients:

- 1 medium onion, chopped
- 1 clove garlic, minced
- 1 small stalk celery, chopped
- ½ pound 93% lean ground beef
- ½ cup low fat evaporated milk
- 1 ½ cups chicken broth, divided
- 4 ounces low fat Velveeta cheese, cubed
- Salt to taste
- ¼ teaspoon paprika to taste
- 1 tablespoon all-purpose flour
- A dozen tortilla chips, crumbled
- Cooking spray

Method:

1. Place a skillet over medium heat. Spray with cooking spray.
2. Add onion, garlic and celery and sauté until translucent.
3. Spray the inside of the slow cooker with cooking spray. Transfer the sautéed onions into it.
4. Place the skillet back on heat and add beef. Cook until the beef is brown. Break it simultaneously as it cooks. Transfer into the slow cooker.
5. Mix together in bowl flour and a little broth and add it to the skillet.
6. Place the skillet back on heat. Add the remaining broth and stir constantly until thick. Scrape any brown bits that were stuck to the bottom of the skillet.
7. Transfer into the slow cooker. Add cheese, salt, pepper and evaporated milk and stir.
8. Cover and set on 'Low' for 2 hours.
9. Ladle into soup bowls. Top with tortilla chips and serve.

Pork Chops with Potatoes

Cooking time: 4 hours

Serves: 2

Smart points: 6

Calories: 267, Carbohydrate – 22 g, Fiber – 3 g, Sugar – 3 g, Fat – 11 g, Protein – 20 g

Ingredients:

- 2 center cut bone in pork chops, trimmed of excess fat
- 2 cloves garlic, crushed
- ½ teaspoon ground cumin
- ¾ teaspoon sazon
- 1 tablespoon all-purpose unbleached flour
- Kosher salt to taste
- Pepper to taste
- 4 ounce Yukon gold potato, peeled, diced
- 4 ounces canned tomato sauce
- ½ red bell pepper, chopped
- 2 tablespoons green pimento olives
- 1 bay leaf
- 3 tablespoons fresh cilantro, chopped

Method:

1. Rub the pork chops with garlic. Mix together in a bowl, sazon, cumin, pepper and salt and rub it over the pork. Sprinkle flour over it and place in the slow cooker.
2. Place tomatoes and red pepper over it. Pour tomato sauce over it. Add about ¼ cup water and bay leaf.
3. Sprinkle olives, half the cilantro and garlic.
4. Cover and cook on 'Low' for 8 hours.
5. Discard the bay leaf.

Garnish with remaining cilantro and serve hot

Chili Beef Slow Cooker

Cooking time: 4-5 hours

Serves: 6

Smart points: 4

Calories: 138, Carbohydrate – 17 g, Fiber – 5 g, Sugar – 2 g, Fat – 3 g, Saturated fat – 1 g Protein – 17 g

Ingredients:

- ½ pound extra lean ground beef or turkey
- 1 medium green bell pepper, deseeded, diced
- 1 medium red bell pepper, deseeded, diced
- 1 teaspoon garlic, minced
- 14 ounces canned crushed tomatoes
- 2 tablespoons canned diced green chilies or 1 small jalapeño pepper, sliced
- 7.5 ounces canned kidney beans, drained, rinsed
- 1 teaspoon ground cumin
- 1 tablespoon chili powder
- 1 small onion, chopped
- Salt to taste
- Pepper to taste
- 1 tablespoon tomato paste

Method:

1. Place a skillet over medium heat. Add beef and garlic and sauté until brown. Break it simultaneously as it cooks. Add bell peppers and sauté for a couple of minutes. Add cumin and chili powder and stir.
2. Transfer into the slow cooker. Add rest of the ingredients and stir well.
3. Cover and cook on 'High' for 4-5 hours.
4. Ladle into bowls and serve.

Slow Cook Chicken chili

Cooking time: 6-8 hours

Serves: 4

Smart points: 5

Calories: 160, Carbohydrate – 24 g, Fiber – 6 g, Sugar – 7 g, Fat – 2 g, Protein – 14 g

Ingredients:

- 6 ounces chicken breast, skinless, boneless, cubed
- 7.5 ounces canned kidney beans, drained
- 7.5 ounces canned corn with its liquid
- 1 cup canned diced tomatoes
- 1 small green bell pepper, chopped
- ¼ cup salsa
- 1 small onion, chopped
- Salt to taste
- Cooking spray

Method:

1. Place a nonstick skillet over medium heat. Spray with cooking spray. Add chicken and cook until brown. Transfer into the slow cooker.
2. Add rest of the ingredients and stir.
3. Cover and cook on 'Low' for 6-8 hours.

Smoothie & Deserts Recipes

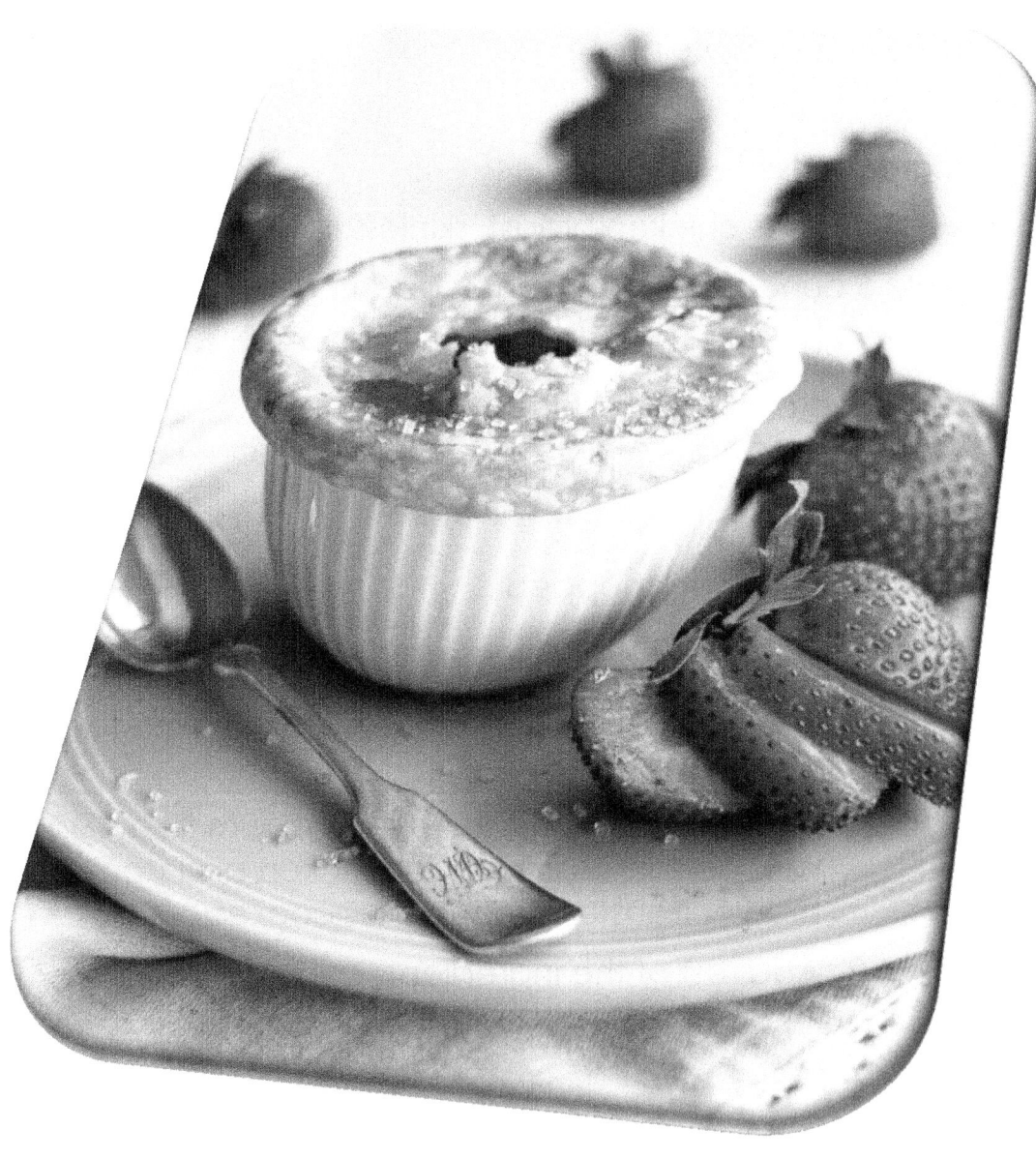

Pineapple & Lemon Smoothie

Serves: 2

Smart points: 1

Calories: 118, Carb 31 g, Fiber 5 g, Sugar 18 g, Protein 2 g,

Ingredients:

- 1 English cucumber, chopped
- 1 ½ cups coconut water
- 4 cups fresh pineapple, frozen
- 2 bunches flat leaf parsley, use only the leaves
- 4 medium lemons, peeled, deseeded, roughly chopped
- 10 drops stevia or to taste

Method:

1. Add all the ingredients into a blender and blend until smooth.
2. Pour into tall glasses and serve.
3. If the pineapples are not frozen, then add ice cubes while blending or crushed ice while serving.

Chia Watermelon Fresca

Serves: 2

Smart points: 2

Calories: 133, Carb 22 g, Sugar 15 g, Fat 6 g Protein 5 g,

Ingredients:

- 3 cups watermelon cubes, deseeded
- 2 tablespoons chia seeds

- 2 slices lemon to garnish
- 1/3 cup water
- 2 sprigs mint to garnish
- Crushed ice to serve

Method:

1. Add all the ingredients into a blender and blend until smooth.
2. Pour into tall glasses and place crushed ice.
3. Garnish with lemon slices and mint sprigs and serve.

Banana Pina Colada Smoothie

Serves: 2

Smart points: 4

Calories: 160, Carb 27 g, Sugar 18 g, Fat 6 g, Protein 2 g

Ingredients:

- 1 medium ripe banana, sliced, frozen
- 1 cup fresh pineapple pieces
- 12 ounces almond coconut milk
- 2 tablespoons chia seeds (optional)
- Ice as required
- 2 tablespoons shredded coconut, sweetened

Method:

1. Add all the ingredients except coconut into a blender and blend until smooth.
2. Pour into tall glasses. Garnish with coconut and serve.

Bali Banana Date Smoothie

Serves: 2

Smart points: 6

Calories: 195, Carb 39 g, Sugar 31 g, Fat 1 g, Protein 5 g

Ingredients:

- 2 dates, pitted, chopped
- 1 medium ripe banana, peeled, sliced
- 1 cup 1% milk
- ½ cup nonfat Greek yogurt
- ¼ teaspoon ground cinnamon
- 1 tablespoon honey
- Ice as required

Method:

1. Add all the ingredients into a blender and blend until smooth.
2. Pour into tall glasses and serve.

Peanut Butter Green Smoothie

Serves: 2

Smart points: 5

Calories: 188, Carb 21 g, Sugar 8.5 g, Fat 11 g, Protein 6g

Ingredients:

- 1 ripe banana, peeled, sliced frozen
- 2 cups baby spinach
- 2 heaping tablespoons cacao nibs
- 4 teaspoons peanut butter
- 1 ½ cups vanilla almond milk, unsweetened

- Stevia drops to taste (optional)
- Ice as required

Method:

1. Add all the ingredients into a blender and blend until smooth.
2. Pour into tall glasses and serve.
3.

Kale, and Hemp Super Smoothie

Serves: 2

Smart points: 2

Calories: 220, Carb 30 g, Sugar 14 g, Fat 10 g, Protein 8 g,

Ingredients:

- 1 cup baby kale
- 1 medium ripe banana, peeled, sliced
- 2 dates, pitted, chopped
- 2 tablespoons raw hemp seeds or any other seeds of your choice
- 1 ½ cups vanilla almond milk, unsweetened
- Ice as required

Method:

1. Add all the ingredients into a blender and blend until smooth.
2. Pour into tall glasses and serve.

Blueberry Kale Smoothie

Serves: 2

Smart points: 5

Calories: 312, Carb 51 g, Sugar 31 g, Fat 12 g, Protein 9 g,

Ingredients:

- 2 cups baby kale
- 1 ½ cups frozen blueberries
- 1 medium ripe banana, peeled, sliced
- 4 dates, pitted, chopped
- 2 tablespoons peanut butter
- 1 ½ cups vanilla almond milk, unsweetened
- Ice as required

Method:

1. Add all the ingredients into a blender and blend until smooth.
2. Pour into tall glasses and serve.

Almond & Berry Smoothie

Serves: 2

Smart points: 4

Calories: 222, Carb 29 g, Sugar 8 g, Fat 11 g, Protein 6 g,

Ingredients:

- 1 ½ cups fresh strawberries, sliced
- 1 ½ cups blueberries, frozen
- 2 tablespoons peanut butter
- 1 ½ cups vanilla almond milk, unsweetened
- Stevia drops to taste

- Ice as required

Method:

1. Add all the ingredients into a blender and blend until smooth.
2. Pour into tall glasses and serve.

Breakfast Oatmeal Smoothie

Serves: 4

Smart points: 5

Calories: 180, Carb 38 g, Sugar 8 g, Fat 2 g, Protein 3 g,

Ingredients:

- 1 cup quick cooking oats, raw
- 1 medium banana, ripe, peeled, sliced
- 1 cup blueberries
- 4 cups water
- 4 tablespoons sugar
- 1 cup almond milk, unsweetened
- Ice as required

Method:

1. Add all the ingredients into a blender and blend until smooth.
2. Pour into tall glasses and serve.
3.

Roasted Strawberry Protein Smoothie

Serves: 2

Smart points: 4

Calories: 213, Carbohydrate – 33 g, Fiber – 7.5 g, Sugar – 27 g, Fat – g, Protein – 16 g.

Ingredients:

- 3 cups fresh strawberries, quartered
- 2/3 cup low fat cottage cheese
- 1 tablespoon sugar
- 1 cup fat free milk
- Stevia drops to taste (optional)
- 2 teaspoons chia seeds

Method:

1. Mix together in a bowl strawberries and sugar. Transfer on to a baking sheet that is lined with parchment paper.

2. Bake in a preheated 425° F for about 15 minutes or until the strawberries begin to release the juices. Remove from the oven and cool for a while. Transfer into a blender.

3. Add rest of the ingredients into the blender and blend until smooth.

4. Pour into tall glasses and serve with crushed ice.

5.

Berry Tartlet with Chocolate & Cream

Cooking time: 12 minutes

Serves: 6   Smart points: 5

Calories: 124, Carbohydrate – 16 g, Fiber – 1 g, Sugar – 10g, Fat – 6.5 g, Protein – 1 g,

Ingredients:

- 5 whole Graham cracker sheets, broken
- 1 tablespoon brown sugar, unpacked
- A pinch kosher salt
- ½ teaspoon sugar
- ¾ ounce dark chocolate, melted
- ¼ teaspoon vanilla extract
- 1 cup mixed berries
- 1 small egg white
- 1 ½ tablespoons unsalted butter, melted, cooled
- 2 tablespoons heavy whipping cream
- Chocolate shavings to garnish (optional)

Method:

1. Line 6 muffin cups with disposable paper liners. Set aside.

2. Add crackers into a food processor and pulse until you get fine crumbs.

3. Mix together in a bowl, crumbs, egg white, salt, butter and brown sugar until well combined. Divide and place this mixture in the muffin cups. Press well to the bottom of the cup.

4. Bake in a preheated oven at 325° F for about 10-12 minutes or a knife when inserted in the center comes out clean. Rotate the pan half way through baking.

5. Meanwhile add cream, sugar and vanilla into a bowl. Whisk with a wire whisk until peaks are formed. Chill for about 5 minutes.

6. Melt the chocolate either in a double boiler or in a microwave.

7. Remove muffin cups from the oven and cool completely. Carefully remove the liner and discard it.

8. Divide and pour the chocolate in the crusts. Freeze the crusts for about 30 minutes.

9. Divide and place berries in the crusts. Spoon some whipped cream. Sprinkle chocolate shavings on top and serve.

Chocolate Cheesecake Cups

Cooking time: 50 minutes

Serves: 6

Smart points: 3

Calories: 65, Carb 6 g, Sugar 6 g, Fat 4 g, Protein 1.5 g

Ingredients:

- 1 small egg

- ½ ounce semisweet baking chocolate + extra shavings to garnish

- 2 tablespoons sugar

- 2 ounces 1/3 less fat cream cheese, softened

- 2 tablespoons light sour cream

Method:

1. Line mini muffin cups with cupcake liners.

2. Melt the chocolate either in a microwave or in a double boiler.

3. Add cream cheese and sugar to a bow. Beat with a hand mixer. Add sour cream and continue beating until smooth.

4. Add egg and fold gently with a spoon. Add melted chocolate and stir until well combined.

5. Place about 2 tablespoons of the mixture in each muffin cup.

6. Bake in a preheated oven at 225° F for about 50 minutes.

7. Once baked, let it remain in the oven for about 30 minutes.

8. Remove from the oven and cool completely.

9. Chill for a few hours. Sprinkle the chocolate shavings over it and serve.

Lemon and Ginger Ice Pops

Cooking time: 5 minutes

Serves: 5

Smart points: 4

Calories: 62, Carbohydrate – 16 g, Fiber – 0 g, Sugar – 15 g, Fat – 0 g, Protein – 0 g,

Ingredients:

- ½ ounce fresh ginger, peeled, minced

- 6 tablespoons sugar
- Zest of 1 ½ lemons, grated
- 1 ¾ cups water
- 2 ½ tablespoons lemon juice
- 5 ultra-thin half lemon slices (optional)

Method:

1. Add ginger, water, sugar and lemon zest to a small saucepan and place on medium heat. Simmer until the sugar is completely dissolved. Remove from heat and cool thoroughly.

2. Pass the mixture through a fine mesh strainer. Press had with the back of the spoon. Add lemon juice and stir.

3. Pour into ice pop molds. Do not fill right up to the top of the mold. Place a slice of lemon in each. Insert Popsicle sticks in each and place in the freezer until set.

Coconut Lime Raspberry Chia Pudding

Serves: 4

Smart points: 5

Calories: 157, Carbohydrate – 15 g, Fiber – 0 g, Sugar – 1 g, Fat – 10 g, Protein – 4 g

Ingredients:

- 1 cup light coconut milk
- 2 cups raspberries
- 4 tablespoons chia seeds
- 1 cup almond coconut milk, unsweetened
- 2 tablespoons shredded coconut, sweetened

- 2 teaspoons lime zest
- 2 teaspoons lime juice
- 15-16 drops stevia drops or to taste

Method:

1. Retain half the raspberries and mix the remaining raspberries with rest of the ingredients in a bowl. Cover and chill for 5-6 hours.

2. Divide the mixture into 4 serving bowls. Divide the raspberries that were set-aside over it and serve.

Dark Chocolate & Nut Clusters Sea Salt

Serves: 10

Smart points: 2

Calories: 54, Carbohydrate – 3 g, Fiber – 0.5 g, Sugar – 2 g, Fat – 5 g, Protein – 1 g

Ingredients:

- 10 pecan halves
- 10 almonds
- 10 walnut halves
- Sea salt as required
- ½ package Ghirardelli dark chocolate melting wafers

Method:

1. Melt the chocolate either in a double boiler or in a microwave.

2. Pick a walnut with a fork and dip into the melted chocolate. Shake off the excess chocolate and place on a tray lined with wax paper. Repeat this procedure with the pecan and place the

dipped pecan over the walnut. Finally repeat this procedure with the almond and place over the pecan. This makes one cluster. Sprinkle a few grains of salt over it.

3. Repeat the above process with the remaining nuts and chocolate. Makes 10 clusters in all.

Candy Corn Fruit Parfaits

Serves: 4

Smart points: 3

Calories: 151, Carb 23 g, Sugar 21 g, Fat 6 g, Protein 3 g

Ingredients:

For the lighter whipped topping:

- ¼ cup heavy whipping cream, chilled
- ¼ cup fat free plain Greek yogurt
- 1 tablespoon sugar
- ¼ teaspoon vanilla

For parfaits:

- 1 1/3 cups jarred mandarin oranges, drained
- 1 1/3 cups diced pineapple (canned or fresh)

Method:

1. Add sugar, vanilla, and cream into a bowl and beat with a chilled hand beater until stiff peaks are formed.
2. Add yogurt and fold.
3. Layer in parfait glasses using mandarin oranges, pineapple and whipped cream.
4. Chill for a while and serve.

Pumpkin Cheesecake Shooters

Serves: 8

Smart points: 3

Calories: 78, Carbohydrate – 11.6 g, Fiber – 0 g, Sugar – 7.5 g, Fat – 4.2 g, Protein – 1 g

Ingredients:

- 0.75 ounces chocolate Graham crackers
- ¼ cup pure canned pumpkin
- 2 ounces 1/3 fat cream cheese, softened
- ½ teaspoon vanilla extract
- ½ teaspoon pumpkin pie spice
- 4 ounces light whipped topping
- 1 ½ tablespoons dark brown sugar, unpacked
- 1/8 teaspoon ground cinnamon
- 1/8 teaspoon ground nutmeg

Method:

1. Place the crackers in a food processor and pulse until crumb like texture is formed. Set aside for a while.
2. Add cream cheese into a bowl and beat with an electric mixer until smooth.
3. Add vanilla, sugar, pumpkin, pumpkin pie spice, cinnamon and nutmeg and beat until smooth and creamy.
4. Add about 2.5 ounces of the whipped topping and mix well. Transfer into a piping bag.
5. Take 8 shot glasses. Sprinkle about ½ teaspoon of cracker crumbs at the bottom of each shot glass.
6. Pipe out some of the pumpkin mixture over it. Dot with a little whipped topping (about a teaspoon).
7. Repeat the above layer once. Finally top with some crumbs.
8. Chill and serve later.

Strawberry Romanoff

Serves: 10

Smart points: 2

Calories: 79, Carbohydrate – 15 g, Fiber – 2 g, Sugar – 12 g, Fat –3 g, Protein – 1 g

Ingredients:

- 32 ounces strawberries, rinsed, cut
- 4 tablespoons brown sugar
- 8 ounce low fat sour cream

Method:

1. Add sour cream and brown sugar into a bowl and mix until brown sugar dissolves.
2. Take 10 glasses. Divide and place the strawberries in the glasses. Spoon in about 2 tablespoons of the sour cream mixture.
3. Chill and serve.

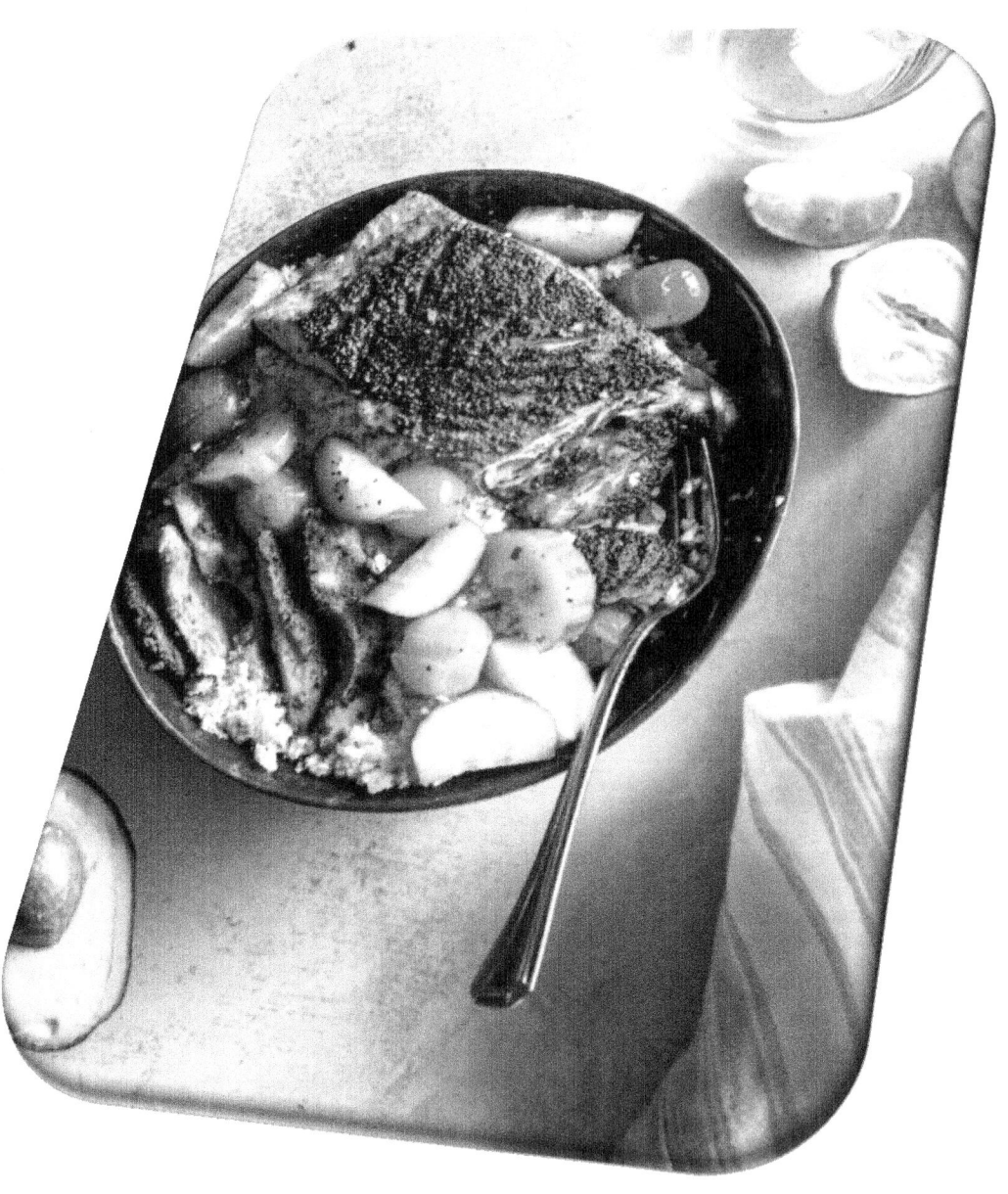

Grilled Salmon Kebabs

Cooking time: 10 minutes

Serves: 2

Smart points: 5

Calories: 267, Carbohydrate – 7 g, Fiber – 3 g, Sugar – 0 g, Fat – 11 g, Protein – 35 g

Ingredients:

- ¾ pound wild salmon fillet, skinless, chopped into 1 inch pieces
- ½ teaspoon ground cumin
- 1 tablespoon fresh oregano, chopped
- ¼ teaspoon red pepper flakes
- 1 teaspoon sesame seeds
- 1 lemon sliced into thin rounds
- kosher salt to taste
- Olive oil cooking spray
- 8 bamboo skewers soaked in water for an hour

Method:

1. Preheat the grill to medium heat. Spray the grill grates with cooking spray.
2. Mix together in a bowl, cumin, red pepper, sesame and oregano and set aside.
3. Thread the salmon on to the skewers with the lemon slices in between.
4. Place the skewers on the grill and grill until the fish turns opaque.
5. Serve hot.

Fettuccini with Poached Eggs

Cooking time: 30 minutes

Serves: 4

Smart points: 8

Calories: 342, Carb 51g, Sugar 2 g, Fat 9 g, Protein 16 g

Ingredients:

- 8 cups wintergreens like chard, spinach, kale etc.
- 8 ounces egg fettuccini
- 1 red onion, thinly sliced
- 4 eggs
- 1 tablespoon olive oil
- 2 cloves garlic, chopped
- 2 sprigs fresh thyme, use only the leaves
- Fresh parmesan cheese, shaved to serve (optional)

Method:

1. Cook the pasta according to the instructions on the package until al dente. Retain about 2 cups of the cooked water and drain the rest.
2. To poach eggs: Place a deep skillet over medium heat. Pour enough water to fill about 2 inches from the bottom of the skillet. Bring to the boil.
3. Lower heat. Crack an egg into a bowl and gently slide it into the water. Similarly repeat with the remaining eggs. Cook the eggs according to the way you like the eggs set. Remove the eggs with a slotted spoon and place over paper towels.
4. Place a large pan over medium high heat. Add oil. When the oil is heated, add onions and salt and sauté until brown. Add garlic and thyme and sauté until fragrant.
5. Add greens and some of the retained cooking water. Cook until the greens wilts.
6. Add pasta and heat thoroughly. Add salt and pepper and stir.

Tasty Potato Gratin

Cooking time: 50 minutes

Serves: 4

Smart points: 6

Calories: 160.2, Carbohydrate – 24.6 g, Fiber – 1.8 g, Sugar – 2.6 g, Fat – 4.4 g,

Protein – 7.2 g

Ingredients:

- 4 medium Yukon gold potatoes (around 1.4 ounces), peeled, cut into 1/8 inch thick slices
- 1 ½ tablespoons butter, melted
- ½ teaspoon garlic powder
- 2 ounces low fat cheddar cheese, shredded
- Salt to taste
- 1 bay leaf
- Freshly ground black pepper to taste
- ¾ cup fat free milk
- 1 teaspoon thyme
- A pinch freshly grated nutmeg
- Cooking spray

Method:

1. Spray a baking dish with cooking spray.
2. Mix together in a bowl, potatoes, garlic powder, salt, pepper and butter. Place half the potatoes in the baking dish. Sprinkle half the cheese.
3. Place the remaining potatoes over it.
4. Place a small saucepan over medium heat. Add milk, thyme, bay leaf and nutmeg and stir. Bring to the boil. Pour this mixture over the potatoes.
5. Sprinkle remaining cheese.
6. Bake in a preheated oven at 425° F for about 45 minutes or until potatoes are cooked.

Eggplant "Meatballs"

Cooking time: 45 minutes

Serves: 12 (4 meatballs each)

Smart points: 6

Calories: 222, Carb 31 g, Sugar 6 g, Fat 7.5 g, Protein 10 g

Ingredients:

- 2 ½ pounds eggplant, unpeeled, cut into 1 inch pieces
- 1 tablespoon olive oil
- 4 cloves garlic, crushed
- 2 large eggs, beaten
- Freshly ground black pepper
- Kosher salt to taste
- 3 cups Italian seasoned breadcrumbs
- 4 ounces Pecorino Romano cheese, freshly grated
- 4 tablespoons fresh basil, chopped + extra to garnish
- 2 tablespoons flat leaf parsley, chopped
- 2 jars (25.25 ounces each) Delallo Pomodoro sauce
- Cooking spray
- Part skim ricotta cheese to serve (optional)

Method:

1. Take a rimmed baking sheet and spray it with cooking spray. Set aside.
2. Place a nonstick skillet over medium high heat. Add oil. When the oil is heated, add eggplant, salt, pepper, and about ½ cup water. Stir occasionally. Cook until tender. Remove from heat and cool for a few minutes.
3. Transfer into a food processor and pulse for a few seconds until well combined.
4. Transfer into a bowl. Add breadcrumbs, salt, pepper, egg, Romano cheese, garlic, parsley and basil. Mix well.
5. Divide and make 48 balls. Roll it tightly and place on the baking sheet that was set aside.
6. Bake in a preheated oven at 375° F until brown and firm.
7. Pour sauce into a skillet and heat. Add the meatballs into the skillet and simmer for 5-6 minutes.
8. Garnish with basil and top with ricotta if desired.

Lighter Baked Macaroni and Cheese

Cooking time: 25

Serves: 4

Smart points: 10

Calories: 269.7, Carb 34.5 g, Fiber 5.3, Protein 15.8 g

Ingredients:

- 6 ounces high fiber elbow pasta
- 2 teaspoons light butter
- 2 teaspoons butter
- 2 tablespoons onion, minced
- 2 tablespoons flour
- ½ cup fat free chicken broth
- 2 cups baby spinach
- 4 ounces 2% reduced fat mild cheddar
- 1 cup skim milk
- Salt to taste
- Pepper to taste
- 2 tablespoons seasoned whole wheat crumbs
- Cooking spray

Method:

1. Cook pasta according to the instructions on the package.
2. Grease a baking dish with butter-flavored pam.
3. Place a heavy skillet over low heat. Add flour and sauté for a few seconds. Add onions and sauté for a couple of minutes.
4. Add milk and chicken broth and stir. Raise the heat to medium high. Stir constantly until thick. Add salt and pepper. Remove from heat.
5. Add cheese and stir until the cheese melts. Add salt and pepper and stir.
6. Add pasta and spinach and stir. Transfer into the prepared baking dish.
7. Sprinkle cheese and breadcrumbs over it.

8. Bake in a preheated oven at 375° F for 15-20 minutes or until the top is golden brown.

Enchiladas Verdes (Green Enchiladas)

Cooking time: 50 minutes

Serves: 4 (2 enchiladas each)

Smart points: 5

Calories: 210, Carbohydrate – 27.5g, Fiber – 3 g, Sugar – 4.5 g, Fat – 4 g, Saturated fat – 0.5 g, Protein – 15 g

Ingredients:

- 1 pound chicken breasts, skinless, boneless
- 1 ½ cups salsa Verde (refer previous chapter for recipe)
- 8 white corn tortillas
- 1 small onion, halved, divided
- ½ cup Queso fresco, crumbled
- Kosher salt to taste
- Fresh cilantro, chopped to garnish
- Sour cream to garnish

Method:

1. Place chicken in a pot filled with water. Place the pot over medium high heat. Add half the onion and salt and stir. Bring to the boil. Simmer until thoroughly cooked.
2. Remove the chicken with a slotted spoon. Shred the chicken with a pair of forks. Set aside for a while.
3. Mince the other half of the onion and add to the chicken.
4. Warm the tortillas according to the instructions on the package. Dip each tortilla in the salsa. Place about 2 tablespoons of the chicken in each tortilla. Roll and place with its seam side down in a single layer in a casserole.
5. Pour the remaining sauce all over the tortillas. Sprinkle Queso fresco.

6. Place the casserole dish in a preheated oven and bake at 400° F for about 20-30 minutes.
7. Garnish with cilantro and sour cream and serve.

Pumpkin Banana Pecan Bread

Cooking time: 50

Serves: 12

Smart points: 4

Calories: 146, Carbohydrate –27 g, Fiber – 2 g, Sugar – 16 g, Fat – 5 g, Protein – 3 g

Ingredients:

- 1 ¼ cups white whole wheat or all-purpose gluten free flour
- ¾ teaspoon pumpkin spice
- 2 tablespoons butter, softened
- ¾ cup pumpkin puree
- ¼ cup apple sauce, unsweetened
- 1.5 ounces pecans, chopped
- ¾ teaspoon baking soda
- ½ teaspoon ground cinnamon
- ¼ teaspoon salt
- ½ cup light brown sugar, not packed
- 2 small ripe bananas, mashed
- 2 large egg whites
- ½ teaspoon vanilla extract
- Cooking spray

Method:

1. Grease a loaf pan with cooking spray.

2. Mix together in a bowl, all the dry ingredients.

3. Add butter and sugar into a large bowl. Beat with an electric mixer until creamy. Add whites, bananas, pumpkin puree, vanilla extract and applesauce. Beat until thick on medium speed. Scrape the sides of the bowl frequently.

4. Add the dry ingredient mixture and pecans and mix on low speed until well combined but not over mixed.

5. Pour the batter into the loaf pan.

6. Bake in a preheated oven 375° F for about 50 minutes or a knife when inserted in the center comes out clean.

Sicilian Rice Ball Casserole

Cooking time: 50
Serves: 4
Smart points: 10
Calories: 373, Carbohydrate – 47 g, Fiber – 2 g, Sugar – 1 g, Fat – 10 g, Saturated fat – 4 g, Protein – 21 g

Ingredients:
- 1 cup long grain rice, uncooked
- 1 ¼ ounces sweet Italian sausage link, casing removed
- 1 small onion, minced
- 2.5 ounces frozen peas
- 5 ounces 93% lean ground turkey
- 1 small egg
- 1 small egg white
- Kosher salt to taste
- Pepper to taste
- 1 cup tomato sauce
- ¾ cup mozzarella cheese
- 4 tablespoons breadcrumbs

- Cooking spray

Method:
1. Cook rice with salt following the instructions on the package. Set aside.
2. Place a skillet over medium heat. Add sausage. Sauté until brown. Break it simultaneously as it cooks.
3. Add turkey and onions and onions and sauté until brown. Break it simultaneously as it cooks.
4. Add salt, pepper, ½ the sauce and peas. Stir.
5. Lower heat, cover and cook for 20 minutes.
6. Mix together in bowl, cooked rice, cheese, egg, egg white, remaining sauce and stir. The mixture will turn out to be slightly sticky.
7. Spray a casserole dish with cooking spray. Sprinkle about 2 tablespoons breadcrumbs on the bottom as well as the sides of the dish.
8. Spread half the rice mixture in the dish. Press well. Layer with half the meat mixture. Sprinkle half the mozzarella.
9. Spread the remaining rice over it, followed by the remaining meat mixture. Next layer with breadcrumbs and remaining mozzarella.
10. Cover the dish with a foil.
11. Bake in a preheated oven at 325° F for about 20 minutes.
12. Garnish with parsley. Chop into wedges and serve.

Chicken and Broccoli Noodle Casserole

Cooking time: 45 minutes

Serves: 3

Smart points: 8

Calories: 313, Carbohydrate – 31.2 g, Fiber – 4.4 g, Sugar – 2.6 g, Fat – 9.9 g, Protein – 27.2 g

Ingredients:
- 3 ounces Ronzoni Smart taste noodles (or no yolk)
- 2 cloves garlic, thinly sliced
- 2 teaspoons butter
- 1 ½ tablespoons all-purpose flour
- ½ cup 1% milk
- 2 ounces reduced fat Sharp cheddar cheese, shredded
- 1 ½ tablespoons parmesan cheese, shredded
- 1 teaspoon oil
- 6 ounces fresh broccoli florets, chopped
- 1 small shallot, minced
- 2/3 cups fat free chicken broth
- 6 ounces cooked shredded chicken breast
- Cooking spray
- 1 tablespoon seasoned bread crumbs

Method:
1. Cook the noodles according to the instructions on the package until al dente (preferably undercooked)
2. Place a skillet over medium heat. Add oil. When the oil is heated, add garlic and sauté until golden brown. Add broccoli and salt and stir.
3. Cover and cook until the broccoli is slightly tender. Remove from heat and set aside.
4. Spray a small casserole dish with cooking spray and set aside.
5. Place a skillet over medium low heat. Add butter. When the butter melts, add shallots and sauté until translucent. Add flour and salt and stir for a couple of minutes on low heat.
6. Add chicken broth and whisk until well combined. And milk and stir. Stir constantly until it thickens.

7. Remove from heat and add cheddar cheese and half the Parmesan and mix until cheese melts. Add chicken, noodles, and broccoli and mix until well coated.
8. Transfer into the prepared casserole dish.
9. Sprinkle remaining Parmesan and breadcrumbs. Spray a little cooking spray.
10. Bake in a preheated oven at 325° F for about 20 – 25 minutes. Broil for a couple of minutes if your want a brown top.

Sloppy Joe Styled Baked Sweet Potatoes

Cooking time: 15

Serves: 2

Smart points: 8

Calories: 259, Carb 40 g, Sugar 4 g, Fat 4 g, Protein 15.5 g,

Ingredients:

- 2 medium sweet potatoes, wash and dry them
- 1 small carrot, chopped
- 4 mushrooms, chopped
- ¼ pound ground beef (93% lean)
- 1 tablespoon red bell pepper, chopped
- 1 clove garlic, minced
- 1 teaspoon Worcestershire sauce
- 12 teaspoon seasoned salt or more to taste
- 1 teaspoon red wine vinegar
- 4 ounces canned tomato sauce
- 3 tablespoons water
- 1 scallion, chopped to garnish
- 1 teaspoon tomato paste

Method:

1. Prick the sweet potatoes all over with a fork. Cook in a microwave until tender.

2. Place a skillet over medium high heat. Add meat and seasoning salt and cook until brown. Break it simultaneously as it cooks.
3. Add onions and garlic and sauté for a couple of minutes. Add carrots, red pepper and mushrooms and sauté for another 3-4 minutes.
4. Lower heat, add vinegar and Worcestershire sauce and cook for 3-4 minutes. Add tomato paste, tomato sauce and water and stir.
5. Cover and simmer until the vegetables are tender.
6. To serve: Cut open the sweet potatoes. Season with salt. Place some of the meat filling on top. Garnish with scallion and serve.

Quick Mexican Brown Rice

Cooking time: 30 minutes

Serves: 3

Smart points: 5

Calories: 200, Carbohydrate – 39 g, Fiber – 3 g, Sugar – 2 g, Fat – 3.5 g, Protein – 5 g

Ingredients:
- 2 cups frozen or cooked brown rice
- 1 medium plum tomato, diced
- 1 clove garlic, minced
- 1 small onion, finely chopped
- 1 jalapeño, deseeded, minced
- 1 tablespoon tomato paste
- ¼ teaspoon cayenne pepper
- ¼ teaspoon ground cumin
- Freshly ground black pepper
- ¼ teaspoon smoked paprika
- 1 teaspoon olive oil
- Kosher salt to taste
- Fresh cilantro leaves, chopped to garnish

- Lime wedges to serve

Method:

1. Cook rice according to the instructions on the package and set aside.
2. Place a skillet over medium high heat. Add onions, tomatoes and jalapeño and sauté until slightly soft.
3. Add garlic and sauté until fragrant.
4. Add rest of the ingredients except rice and stir. Add rice and mix well. Heat thoroughly and serve garnished with cilantro and lime wedges.

Quinoa and Spinach Patties

Cooking time:

Serves: 3

Smart points: 6

Calories: 236.2, Carbohydrate – 30.5g, Fiber – 3.2 g, Sugar – 1.9 g, Fat – 7.4 g, Protein – 11.4 g

Ingredients:

- 1 ¼ cups uncooked quinoa, rinsed
- 2 eggs, whisked
- 1 ¼ cups water
- 3 medium scallions, thinly sliced
- 3 tablespoons parmesan cheese, grated
- ½ cup steamed spinach, chopped
- 2 cloves garlic, minced
- Kosher salt to taste
- 1 teaspoon olive oil
- ½ cup plain breadcrumbs

Method:

1. Pour water into a medium saucepan. Add quinoa and stir. Bring to the boil.
2. Lower heat and simmer until tender and all the water has been absorbed. Remove from heat and cool. Transfer into a bowl.

3. Add rest of the ingredients except oil and set aside for a few minutes.
4. Divide the mixture into 6 portions. Form each into patties.
5. Place a nonstick pan over medium heat. Add oil. When the oil is heated, place the patties and cook until the underside is brown. Flip sides and cook the other side is brown too. Cook in batches if necessary.
6. Serve with a dip of your choice.

Tuscan White Beans with Spinach and Shrimp

Cooking time: 15 minutes

Serves: 2

Smart points: 7

Calories: 282, Carbohydrate – 22.2 g, Fiber – 6.2 g, Sugar – 0.2 g, Fat – 6.9g, Protein – 32.5 g

Ingredients:

● ½ pound large shrimp, peeled, deveined (weigh it after peeling)
● 2 cloves garlic, minced
● 1 small onion, chopped
● 1 tablespoon balsamic vinegar
● 1 teaspoon extra virgin olive oil
● 1 teaspoon fresh sage, chopped
● ¼ cup cannellini beans, rinsed, drained
● ¾ ounce reduced fat feta cheese, crumbled

Method:

1. Place a skillet over medium high heat. Add oil. When ½ teaspoon oil. When the oil is heated, add shrimp and cook until it just turns opaque. Transfer into a bowl and set aside.
2. Add the remaining oil to the skillet and heat. Add onions, garlic and sage and sauté until it turns golden brown.

3. Add vinegar and stir. Add broth and stir. Bring to the boil.
4. Add beans and spinach and cook until spinach wilts.
5. Remove from heat and shrimp. Stir well.
6. Divide into bowls. Sprinkle feta cheese on to and serve.

Buffalo Turkey Cheeseburger with Broccoli Slaw

Cooking time: 15 minutes

Serves: 10

Smart points: 8

Calories: 358, Carbohydrate – 22.7 g, Fiber – 5.6 g, Sugar – 5.9 g, Fat – 15 g, Protein – 38.3 g

Ingredients:
- 2 ½ pounds 93% lean ground turkey
- 3 cups broccoli slaw
- 1 1/3 cups carrots, grated
- ½ cup blue cheese dressing
- 2 cloves garlic, grated
- ½ cup seasoned whole wheat breadcrumbs
- 1 tablespoon red onion, grated
- Salt to taste
- Freshly ground pepper to taste
- ½ cup hot sauce or to taste
- 10 slices low fat cheddar
- Cooking spray
- 10 whole wheat burger buns, split

Method:
1. Mix together in a bowl, turkey, breadcrumbs, carrots, onion, garlic, salt, pepper and hot sauce. Divide into 10 portions and shape each portion into a patty.
2. Mix together in a bowl, broccoli slaw and blue cheese dressing and set aside.

3. Place a skillet over high heat. Spray with cooking spray. Place 2-3 patties at a time.
4. Lower heat to medium low. Cook until the bottom side is golden brown. Flip sides and cook the other side too. Cook the burgers in batches.
5. Toast the burger buns. Place a patty over each bun. Top with cheese and broccoli slaw and serve.

FreeStyle 200+ Zero Points Foods

Here it is: an expanded list of all 200+ zero Points foods.* The foods on this list form the foundation of a healthy eating pattern, so you don't need to weigh, measure, or track any of them

Apples
Applesauce, unsweetened
Apricots
Arrowroot
Artichoke hearts
Artichokes
Arugula
Asparagus

Bamboo shoots
Banana
Beans: including adzuki, black, broad (fava), butter, cannellini, cranberry (Roman), green, garbanzo (chickpeas), great northern, kidney, lima, lupini, mung, navy, pink, pinto, small white, snap, soy, string, wax, white
Beans, refried, fat-free, canned
Beets
Berries, mixed
Blackberries
Blueberries
Broccoli
Broccoli rabe
Broccoli slaw
Broccolini

Brussels sprouts

Cabbage: all varieties including Chinese (bok choy), Japanese, green, red, napa, savory, pickled
Calamari, grilled
Cantaloupe
Carrots
Cauliflower
Caviar
Celery
Swiss chard
Cherries
Chicken breast, ground, 99% fat-free
Chicken breast or tenderloin, skinless, boneless or with bone
Clementines
Coleslaw mix (shredded cabbage and carrots), packaged
Collards
Corn, baby (ears), white, yellow, kernels, on the cob
Cranberries
Cucumber

Daikon
Dates, fresh
Dragon fruit

Edamame, in pods or shelled
Egg substitutes
Egg whites
Eggplant
Eggs, whole, including yolks
Endive
Escarole

Fennel (anise, sweet anise, or finocchio)
Figs
Fish: anchovies, arctic char, bluefish, branzino (sea bass), butterfish, carp, catfish, cod, drum, eel, flounder, grouper, haddock, halibut, herring, mackerel, mahimahi (dolphinfish), monkfish, orange roughy, perch, pike, pollack, pompano, rainbow trout (steelhead), rockfish, roe, sablefish (including smoked),

salmon (all varieties), salmon, smoked (lox), sardines, sea bass, smelt, snapper, sole, striped bass, striped mullet, sturgeon (including smoked); white sucker, sunfish (pumpkinseed), swordfish, tilapia, tilefish, tuna (all varieties), turbot, whitefish (including smoked), whitefish and pike (store-bought), whiting

Fish fillet, grilled with lemon pepper

Fruit cocktail

Fruit cup, unsweetened

Fruit salad

Fruit, unsweetened

Garlic

Ginger root

Grapefruit

Grapes

Greens: beet, collard, dandelion, kale, mustard, turnip

Greens, mixed baby

Guavas

Guavas, strawberry

Hearts of palm (palmetto)

Honeydew melon

Jackfruit

Jerk chicken breast

Jerusalem artichokes (sunchokes)

Jicama (yam bean)

Kiwifruit

Kohlrabi

Kumquats

Leeks

Lemon

Lemon zest

Lentils

Lettuce, all varieties

Lime

Lime zest

Litchis (lychees)

Mangoes
Melon balls
Mung bean sprouts
Mung dal
Mushroom caps
Mushrooms: all varieties including brown, button, crimini, Italian,
portabella, shiitake

Nectarine
Nori seaweed

Okra
Onions
Oranges: all varieties including blood

Papayas
Parsley
Passion fruit
Pea shoots
Peaches
Peapods, black-eye
Pears
Peas and carrots
Peas: black-eyed, chickpeas (garbanzo), cowpeas (blackeyes,
crowder, southern), young pods with seeds, green, pigeon, snow
(Chinese pea pods); split, sugar snap
Peppers, all varieties
Pepperoncini
Persimmons
Pickles, unsweetened
Pico de gallo
Pimientos, canned
Pineapple
Plumcots (pluots)
Plums
Pomegranate seeds
Pomegranates
Pomelo (pummelo)
Pumpkin

Pumpkin puree

Radicchio
Radishes
Raspberries
Rutabagas

Salad, mixed greens
Salad, side, without dressing, fast food
Salad, three-bean
Salad, tossed, without dressing
Salsa verde
Salsa, fat free
Salsa, fat free; gluten-free
Sashimi
Satay, chicken, without peanut sauce
Satsuma mandarin
Sauerkraut
Scallions
Seaweed
Shallots
Shellfish: abalone, clams, crab (including Alaska king, blue, dungeness, lump crabmeat, queen) crayfish, cuttlefish, lobster (including spiny lobster), mussels, octopus, oysters, scallops, shrimp, squid
Spinach
Sprouts, including alfalfa, bean, lentil
Squash, summer (all varieties including zucchini)
Squash, winter (all varieties including spaghetti)
Starfruit (carambola)
Strawberries
Succotash

Tangelo
Tangerine
Taro
Tofu, all varieties
Tofu, smoked
Tomatillos
Tomato puree

Tomato sauce
Tomatoes: all varieties including plum, grape, cherry
Turkey breast, ground, 99% fat-free
Turkey breast or tenderloin, skinless, boneless or with bone
Turkey breast, skinless, smoked
Turnips

Vegetable sticks
Vegetables, mixed
Vegetables, stir fry, without sauce

Water chestnuts
Watercress
Watermelon

Yogurt, Greek, plain, nonfat, unsweetened
Yogurt, plain, nonfat, unsweetened
Yogurt, soy, plain

Conclusion

All the recipes given here will assist you further in following the program. You can still eat delicious food while losing weight; it does not have to mean eating tasteless and unfulfilling food. Such approaches will only make you give up on your weight loss goal faster.

So go slow and steady with Weight Watchers and see the results. You can also go ahead and recommend or gift it to anyone that you think could use the help as well.

Lightning Source UK Ltd.
Milton Keynes UK
UKOW05f1928020218
317309UK00005B/150/P

9 781983 625619